THE ECOLOGY OF
MENTAL DISORDER

THE ECOLOGY OF
MENTAL DISORDER

Leo Levy, Ph.D., S.M. hyg.
Associate Professor
University of Illinois at
the Medical Center

Louis Rowitz, Ph.D.
Research Scientist
Illinois State Pediatric Institute
&
Assistant Professor
University of Illinois at
the Medical Center

Behavioral Publications   **New York**
1973

Library of Congress Catalog Number 73-6767
Standard Book Number 87705-034-1
Copyright © 1973 by Behavioral Publications

BEHAVIORAL PUBLICATIONS, 2852 Broadway—Morningside Heights,
New York, New York 10025

Printed in the United States of America
This printing 10 9 8 7 6 5 4 3 2 1

Library of Congress Cataloging in Publication Data

Levy, Leo, 1928-
  The ecology of mental disorder.

  Bibliography: p.
  1. Mentally ill--Chicago. I. Rowitz, Louis,
joint author. II. Title. [DNLM: 1. Ecology.
2. Mental disorders. 3. Mental disorders--Occurrenc
--Chicago. WM 100 L662e 1973]
RC445.I28L48   614.5'8'0977311   73-6767
ISBN 0-87705-034-1

TABLE OF CONTENTS

LIST OF MAPS

LIST OF TABLES

FOREWORD

Epidemiological studies of mental disorder have shown a marked acceleration after World War II. The current study by Levy and Rowitz comes at the end of these fertile decades for epidemiological research of mental illness. The authors take into account many of the previous inconsistent findings of these studies and build upon their increasing methodological sophistication. Indeed Levy and Rowitz have tried to take full advantage of this situation in the following way. They do not direct their efforts to establish relationships between the social environment and incidence rates. Rather, they point to the demographic and social characteristics of areas where many cases of mental illness are found in contrast to these characteristics of areas where few cases are found. Levy and Rowitz speak of high hospital utilization rates by areas rather than of high incidence rates by areas. However, this does not tell the whole story and I shouldn't at this point anticipate their findings.

They started out to replicate the study that Robert Faris and I carried to completion over 30 years ago, but they ended theirs by pointing to the various ways in which their work has significantly differed from the concerns that had guided Faris and myself. Differences in focus and methodology stand out clearly. Nevertheless, the voluminous amount of data, amassed by Levy and Rowitz in their numerous maps and tables (26 maps and 38 tables), will provide some interesting contrasts with comparable data in the Faris-Dunham volume. The contrasts are suggestive of new insights into the interpretation of spatial distribution patterns of the various types of mental illness.

I must confess to a touch of nostalgia in reading the Levy and Rowitz account. For it provided me with a keen sense of having been there before and I felt a resurgence of the excitement that had gripped me at the time when I viewed the final maps showing the distribution of schizophrenic rates in contrast to the distribution of manic-depressive rates in the city of Chicago. It was a period when many pieces of exhilarating empirical sociological research were under way at the University of Chicago and the distribution of schizophrenic rates suggested the possibility that there might be so called "insanity areas" in the city in much the same manner as there existed "delinquency areas" which Clifford Shaw had identified in the previous decade. The random rate distribution of the manic-depressive psychoses only served to tighten the findings concerning the concentration of high rates of schizophrenia at the city's center.

· As I look back at the period I cannot help but wonder if the general *zeitgeist* of an age is not a more significant factor in determining the interpretation often given to social data than are the alternative interpretations logically flowing from the empirical data that have been collected. In other words, the interpretation is made as the *zeitgeist* ordains rather than as the data suggest. In any case, it is clear now after three decades of epidemiological research of mental disorders that our interpretation—even though as Professor Burgess indicated it was congenial to the sociological student—was too hasty and was too much at a variance with the facts and the hidden methodological assumptions as these began to emerge and to be discussed.

Levy and Rowitz are rightly more cautious in their conclusions and, as I indicated above, have attempted to point to the contrasts between the ecological characteristics of high rate areas and these same characteristics for low rate areas. In still another fashion some of their empirical findings support certain recent observations concerning the distribution of mental disorder within the urban environment. I am referring to the distribution of schizophrenic first admission rates which they describe as random and which at all events differ from the highly concentrated rates at the center of the city that Faris and I discovered. As a matter of fact, their frequency distribution of schizophrenic rates forms almost a perfect normal probability curve in contrast to the highly skewed curve—the bulk of the communities with low rates and a half a dozen communities with high rates—that Faris and I reported a generation ago. This finding as much as any has pointed to the changing ecological organization of our cities and emphasizes the naivete in our interpretation of the schizophrenic rate pattern. Thus it is apparent that the rate patterns found by Levy and Rowitz do reflect changing ecological organization of the cities, a new organization which has emerged as a result of human intervention through the new technology, planned urban renewal, the development of urban freeways, the deterioration of the city schools and the unmet rising expectations of the Blacks.

These are some of the factors that have changed the ecological organization of the urban community. Further, it should be noted that a sharp contrast between the distribution of schizophrenic unduplicated admissions and schizophrenic first admissions lends support, as they have noted, to the "drift" hypothesis which, in turn, is an inadequate formulation of the social selection process. Finally, they find that low rate areas are homogeneous in their demographic composition while high rate areas are much more heterogeneous as they contain a diverse demographic mixture of social classes and ethnic groups. This seems to me quite significant and suggests the possibility that poor mental and emotional adjustments of persons tend to flourish amidst cultural diversity, but tend to be abated in a climate of cultural unity.

Professors Levy and Rowitz are to be commended for the caution in their interpretation, the new emphasis apparent in their study, and their attempt to build upon the previous epidemiological studies of mental disorder. Their work should help to bring us closer to an identification of those social factors which may be causative or precipitous with respect to the various mental disorders and also to the identification of those distorted personality types and inadequate emotional adjustments which truly emerge from the social process.

It is my sincere hope that this work will help to enrich our sociological imagination towards the end of understanding and unraveling the infinite ways in which the distortions, disturbances and abnormalities of the human personality are inextricably woven by and into the social process. This is a worthy goal for any ecological study and one that Professors Levy and Rowitz in this study have attempted to achieve.

H. Warren Dunham

School of Medicine
Wayne State University

AUTHORS' PREFACE

While our intellectual debt to Robert E. L. Faris and H. Warren Dunham should be apparent even to the casual reader, it should be pointed out that the present study does not attempt a replication of their pioneering effort reflected in the 1939 publication of *Mental Disorders in Urban Areas*. There are some very important differences both in methodology and focus of interest which clearly differentiate the studies.

1. Faris and Dunham reported first admissions to public and private mental hospitals from Chicago. The present study reports all persons admitted (unduplicated admissions) as well as first admissions to 44 public mental hospitals, private mental hospitals, and psychiatric units of general hospitals from Chicago.

2. Faris and Dunham presented data for the years 1922-1934. The present study reports a single year's admission, the fiscal year 1961 (July 1, 1960—June 30, 1961).

3. The Faris and Dunham data were presented on the basis of both Chicago community area and census tracts. The present study reports only community area breakdowns.

4. The Faris and Dunham study reported the total of first admissions for all diagnostic categories assessed including: schizophrenia (and subtypes), manic-depressive psychosis, senile dementia, general paresis, alcoholism, and drug addiction. The present study reports unduplicated and first admissions for

all diagnostic categories assessed including: schizophrenia (no subtypes), manic-depressive psychosis, diseases of the senium (senile dementia and cerebral arteriosclerosis), alcoholism, and a combined category of psychoneurotic, psychophysiologic, and personality disorders.

5. The ecologic indices employed by Faris and Dunham in the analyses of their community areas were: % Negro; % foreign born; % native white of foreign or mixed parents; % male; % female; % under and over 30 years of age; % 65 years of age and over; ratio of married to single people; education in years; % of home ownership; % of hotel residents and lodging houses; % of families owning radios; % residents; % of juvenile delinquents; and mortality rates. The ecologic indices used in the present study in the analysis of community areas are: % Negro; % foreign born; % native born with one or both parents foreign born; % native born with native parentage; % male; % female; % 18 years of age and under; % 65 years of age and older; % single, married, widowed, separated, and divorced; median school years completed; % with 4 or more years of college; % of workers in manufacturing jobs; % of male white-collar workers; % of labor force unemployed; median family income; % with $3000 annual income or less; % with $10,000 annual income or more; % houses built 1950 or later; % dwellings owner-occupied; % substandard housing; % dwellings with more than one person per room; median value of owner units in one-unit structures; median number of rooms per dwelling; median gross rent for rental units; commitments to the Illinois Youth Commission— juvenile male delinquents 1958-1962; illegitimate births 1962; public assistance recipients 1962; % residents moved since 1955; and average suicide rate 1959-1963.

Differences in Major Foci of Interest between The Two Studies

One of the major thrusts of the Faris and Dunham study was to establish a true incidence figure for mental illness using hospital first admissions. This was not a major concern of the present study, nor were we concerned with establishing an accurate measure of prevalence of major mental disorder.

The principal intent of the present study was to establish the ecological characteristics of communities which produced differential rates of psychiatric casualties. The absolute size of these rates (whether for first or unduplicated admissions), while reported and used to differentiate areas, is nowhere emphasized. When, for example, a high unduplicated admission rate area is designated as one with a rate of 725+ admissions per 100,000 adult population per year, the designation does not carry the implication that this level is high in any absolute sense, nor does it imply that this rate reflects all psychiatric cases potentially countable (say by survey) in the community in question. We know, in fact, that all our reported rates must be underestimates because: a) not all cases of psychiatric disorder are hospitalized or even treated; b) Veteran's Administration admission figures for the period were unavailable; and c) admissions from Chicago to hospitals outside the state were not available. The omissions would constitute potent sources of error if our intent was to establish either true incidence or prevalence rates. Our intent was rather to differentiate areas of the city which generated high and low rates of psychiatric casualties as measured by hospital admissions. Having established this, our next task was to determine if and how these areas, so differentiated, differed along a set of demographic dimensions furnished by the United States Census of 1960 and other sources.

We could not state with any conviction that a low-rate area is in any general sense "mentally healthier" than a high-rate area. Our data only reflects the tendency of persons to come from areas with certain demographic credentials when admitted to an in-patient psychiatric facility. This data, however, coupled with information about diagnoses and the types of facility to which they go, constitutes a vast body of information which the present volume attempts to finally assemble and digest.

Acknowledgements

A study of the magnitude of the present one has been aided at various points by many people. First, it is important to thank the Illinois Department of Mental Health and specifically the statistics section, which carried out the data collection. Thanks must also be given to the many people who contributed their efforts towards the completion of the study. Specifically, we would like to thank Edward D'Elia, Robert Warman, Warren Smith, Allen N. Herzog, Mary Grossberg, Audrey Turner, Ferdinand Runk, Dennis Dylong, Thomas Barrett, Lori Magnusson, V. J. Moses, Toni Rowitz, and Jannette Childress. All these people contributed during various phases and in various ways to the completion of this study.

Special acknowledgement should be given to H. Warren Dunham for his inspiration and kind guidance during the various phases of the research.

1. MENTAL DISORDERS IN URBAN AREAS: A REVIEW OF THE LITERATURE

In 1939, Robert E. L. Faris and H. Warren Dunham published their pioneering study of mental disorder in Chicago. Their study utilized data on all first admissions to public and private mental hospitals from 1922 through 1934 from the seventy-five community areas of Chicago (Faris and Dunham, 1960). They found that areas of high social disorganization located at or near the city center are the areas in which the highest rates of mental illness occur. Specifically they concluded:

1. Mental illness, like other social problems, fits into the ecological structure of the city;[1]

2. The highest rates of schizophrenia are to be found in the "disorganized communities at or near the center of the city." The schizophrenia rate tends to decline in every direction the further one gets from the city center;

3. There is a tendency, although not a very strong one, for the manic-depressive cases to come from the higher socio-economic areas. However, ecological patterns of manic-depressive cases tend to be random;

4. Alcoholic psychoses have their highest rates in or near the city center, as do drug addiction and general paresis rates;

5. While the psychoses of old age show a pattern similar to the schizophrenic rates, the rates do not always

1

show a decline farther away from the center of the city. In brief, these were the main findings of an extremely important study. It was the first systematic foray into a luxuriously rich conceptual area. It had no comparable antecedents and stimulated many studies over the succeeding three decades.

ANTECEDENT STUDIES

Historically, studies of the ecology of mental disorders appeared infrequently in the psychiatric literature. In 1875, P. M. Deas looked at the distribution of insanity in 5 geographic subsections in Cheshire, England (Deas, 1875). He found that there was a greater development of insanity in some geographic areas than in others. In the high insanity areas, in comparison to low rate areas, Deas noted an increasing ratio of insanity among men as compared to women, a large proportion of cases due to organic disease or degeneration, a small ratio of recoveries, and a large proportion of deaths.

A. O. Wright, writing in 1884, noted the differing insanity rates reported in the 1880 census for different regions in the United States. The rate reported for the state of Massachusetts was the highest for any state and the rate declined roughly in proportion to the distance from that state traveling in any direction (Wright, 1884). The author clearly favors the explanation that the more recently settled areas of the country are inhabited by "a selected population, mostly young and middle aged people of sound minds and bodies. The insane are left behind. . ." (Wright, 1884, p. 232).

The same pattern of geographical distribution of insanity from the 1880 and 1890 censuses, analyzed by W. A. White in 1903, elicits a different interpretation. White's view is that the stresses and strains of civilization encourage the development of mental disorder. He states: "The savage in his simplicity does not know what it is to suffer from the cares and worries which are the daily portion of the European, and it is little wonder that the latter, beset by all manner of disappointments and vexations, should more frequently break down in mind than his less gifted brother." (White, 1903, p. 263). This general view leads one to predict higher rates of mental illness in older (and larger) cities than in the frontiers where life is presumed simpler.

Sutherland (1901) noting both the growth in lunacy ratios and differential distribution among the four main areas of Scotland sets out five explanatory propositions listed in order of importance:

1. Economic capacity of householders in different counties to maintain the insane without public assistance;

2. Migration of the strong from rural to urban areas leaves the feeble in the rural areas;

3. High infant mortality in the cities eliminates many lunatics that would survive in a rural setting;

4. Conditions of modern life such as competition, abuse of alcohol and tea, poor diet, etc., set up deranged metabolism and disturb mental equilibrium;

5. The definition of lunacy is being widened and hence there is a widened portal of entry to the official registry as a lunatic.

In an interesting letter to the British Medical Journal in 1908, W. R. MacDermott cites differences in insanity rates for several counties in Ireland which had stable populations (same families for at least 100 years) (MacDermott, 1908). He found increases in insanity in several areas and concluded that environmental factors rather than inheritance accounted for the increase in insanity rates.

At the seventieth annual meeting of the Medico-Psychological Association in Dublin in 1911, Dr. W. R. Dawson gave a presidential address on the relationship between geographical distribution of insanity and certain social conditions in Ireland (Dawson, 1911). He pointed out that insanity is prevalent in agricultural countries and is closely tied to poverty. He saw some correspondence between insanity rates and emigration rates. Some slight relationship existed between mental illness, the prevalence of criminality, and chronic alcoholism. Dawson saw no appreciable relationship between insanity and density of population, valuation of land, or distribution of drunkenness as opposed to alcoholism.

The contributions of these authors are important in that each documents a differential spatial distribution of mental illness. Sutherland raises issues which are still current concerning socio-economic status, migration, and the problem of defining mental illness. His reflections on the strains of modern life along with White's similar observations may be considered romantic and not internally consistent. If, as White states, the more civilized and gifted are more prone to psychological disorder, one must account for the fact that within cities it is the poor and the less-educated who appear to manifest higher rates of mental disorder. It is necessary to note that Dawson found higher rates of insanity in rural areas with a great deal of poverty. Wright's point about the sturdier stock going out to the frontier leaving the aged, the infirm of body and spirit, and other weaker souls would sound reasonable if MacDermott had not found that there was an increase in insanity even in areas with very stable populations. The problem is that Wright does not deal well with the low rates in the southern part of the U. S. which was definitely not the frontier, nor with the fact that rates of insanity increase as one goes west from Colorado to California. He explains these inconsistent findings with an assertion that Negroes are mentally healthier than whites (that disposes of the low rates in the south) and that there are a lot of homeless men subjected to hardships of life in mining and lumbering camps in California. If we could discount Dawson's findings of higher prevalence in agricultural areas, it is interesting that none of the other authors appear to entertain the possibility that the differential rates of mental disorder in urban versus rural areas may be explained by the greater accessibility of psychiatric services at or near the larger and older cities and the higher visibility of deviant behavior in densely populated cities.

STUDIES OF ECOLOGICAL PATTERNING OF MENTAL ILLNESS IN URBAN AREAS

Following hard on the Faris and Dunham study of Chicago, similarly designed studies were executed in St. Louis, Milwaukee, Omaha, Kansas City, Rockford, Peoria, Cleveland, and Providence (Schroeder, 1942; Queen, 1940). The findings with regard to admissions for all diagnoses generally follow the patterning observed by Faris and Dunham in Chicago. Highest rates tended to be clustered about the city center and rates tended to lessen as distance from the city center increased. For individual diagnoses, however, the results differed somewhat from the Chicago pattern. In St. Louis, the schizophrenic rates did not follow the pattern in a conclusive way. In Milwaukee, the schizophrenic rates concentrated in the city center, but tended to extend further out than the admission rates for all diagnoses. In Omaha and Kansas City, the schizophrenic rates with some variation did follow the pattern for all admissions. The results in Peoria were inconclusive because of the small number of cases studied. Cleveland data lent partial support to the hypothesis that institutionalized mental patients came predominantly from areas of dense population, low economic status, and high rates of delinquency, most of which areas surround the central business district. In

Providence, Faris' study of a single public mental hospital yielded results similar to those obtained in Cleveland. Faris and Dunham's findings of a general scattering of admissions for manic-depressive psychosis throughout the city was verified in each of the cities studied. Only the St. Louis study examined admission rates for senile psychosis and found, contrary to the Chicago study, a random pattern of admissions.

Gerard and Houston (1953), studying 305 male first admission schizophrenics to the State Mental Hospital from Worcester, Massachusetts between 1931 and 1950, found a typical ecological distribution of schizophrenia. However, when analyzed by family setting, it was found that the typical ecological pattern is based on the residential pattern of a minority of patients, i.e., the single men living alone. The majority of patients were living in a family setting at the time of admission. These patients were distributed without central concentration. There was greater residential instability for patients living alone at the time of first admission than for those living in family settings. Stein (1957), in a study of first admissions for several diagnoses from two areas of London for the years 1954-55, found higher admission rates from the higher social class west boroughs of London than for the lower class east boroughs. This pattern held for schizophrenia as well as all diagnoses combined. Clausen and Kohn (1959) did not establish spatial patterning in their study of schizophrenics in Hagerstown, Maryland. Specifically, they argue that their data show no apparent relationship between the socio-economic levels of areas of the city and rate of hospitalization for first admissions.

A recent study by Hafner and Reimann (1970), investigating first admissions from the city of Mannheim (Germany), reports topographic distributions of mental disorder similar to that found by Faris and Dunham in Chicago.

What can be gleaned from the multiplicity of studies reviewed to this point? First, it is apparent that the studies differ in quality and design. The area of psychiatric epidemiology is fraught with methodological difficulties which are detailed in an ensuing chapter. It appears that in large urban areas, patterning of admissions to psychiatric hospitals is a fact. The patterning is clear enough for all diagnoses combined but becomes more disputed as separate diagnostic categories are considered. Further, the spatial arrangement of admissions appears to be subordinate to certain broad socio-economic and demographic variables which create the identity of areas. There is nothing inherent in the spatial location of the central city which produces numerous psychiatric casualties. Rather, it is the fact that large cities generally have their poverty concentrated in the city center and poverty abates as one proceeds outwards to the suburbs. This is certainly not a perfect relationship and all large cities are not similar, but the relationship is good enough, apparently, and cities beyond a certain size are similar enough, apparently, to create a series of effects mainly contingent upon the poverty variable.

ISSUES RAISED BY
STUDIES OF
ECOLOGICAL DISTRIBUTION
OF MENTAL DISORDER
IN URBAN AREAS

Aside from serious problems of methodology which will be reviewed later, these studies and others which will be dealt with shortly pose a number of fascinating issues:

1. Are schizophrenia and other mental disorders in any important sense caused by the environment in which a

person is raised? This has come to be referred to by the shorthand phrase "social causation."

2. If schizophrenia and other mental disorders are not in any important sense caused by factors definable as environmental, then are there specifiable processes by which cases aggregate spatially and demographically? This has come to be referred to by the shorthand phrase "social selection."

3. Do measures of incidence and prevalence produce comparable ecological distributions of schizophrenia and other mental disorders? Incidence is generally defined as first admissions, treated prevalence as unduplicated admissions, and prevalence as complete count of disordered persons for an area.

As one can readily understand, these issues strike at the heart of some vital concerns for a number of scientific disciplines and the Faris and Dunham study of Chicago posed the issues in sharp terms. Myerson (1940), in reviewing the study, immediately raised the issue of the "drift hypothesis" (now subsumed under social selection), an issue much discussed to the present. In general, the drift hypothesis holds that persons with schizophrenia, as a result of the illness, drift downwards in the social structure. Measures of the drifting process can be intergenerational or intragenerational. Operationally this would mean demonstrating either a status differential between the father of the schizophrenic and the patient or a status differential in the patient at different points in his life (e.g., at the point of first admission and at some later point). The issue of drift has been applied to schizophrenia, but could as well be applied to any chronic disabling mental illness which has its onset relatively early in the person's life. It turns out, however, that the other categories of psychiatric diagnosis do not meet these specifications as schizophrenia does or is thought to. Manic-depressive psychosis, for example, while possibly chronic, is not disabling except during relatively brief episodes of illness which are thought to be self-limiting with or without treatment. Psychoneurosis, psychosomatic disorders, and personality disorders, while possibly chronic, are for the most part never as disabling as schizophrenia. Senile dementia is chronic and progressively disabling but its onset is too late in life to make a measure of downward drift meaningful. Perhaps alcoholism and possibly other addictions come closest to the criteria of early onset, chronicity, and serious disability which characterize schizophrenia. Indeed, the rapid downward descent of the alcoholic is much more familiar in the popular literature than that of the schizophrenic.

LaPouse, Monk, and Terris (1956) conclude from their two-year study of first admission schizophrenics to two mental hospitals serving the Buffalo (N. Y.) area that the concentration of schizophrenic admissions from low socio-economic areas is not the result of drift of these patients into these areas. They also conclude that the concentration of these patients in low socio-economic areas is not the result of upward mobility of normal persons and the stagnation of schizophrenic patients. Their study is in agreement with earlier data from a study by Hollingshead and Redlich (1954), which found that parents of schizophrenic patients had not been located in higher social classes than their schizophrenic children.

Turner and Wagenfeld (1967), using data from the Monroe County (N. Y.) psychiatric case register, studied a group of 214 schizophrenic first admissions. They conclude that there is indeed intergenerational drift (which they call social selection) and that this factor substantially explains the heavy loadings of schizophrenic patients in the lower occupational categories. Intragenerational drift (which they call social drift) makes only a minor contribution to this finding. Their conclusions are in agreement with Grunfeld and Salvesen (1968) who found a decline intergenerationally in social status in their sample of 85 schizophrenic patients admitted to

Gaustad Hospital (Norway) between 1955 and 1958. A five-year follow-up of these patients compared to a group of 101 reactive psychosis patients showed additional (social) drift.

Dunham has presented arguments in his recent writings to explain the concentration of schizophrenics in the lower socio-economic areas of the city. In *Community and Schizophrenia* (1965) he carefully contrasts two communities in Detroit in which he established the incidence of schizophrenia to differ by a factor of 3. He proceeds to demonstrate that this apparent difference is reduced to insignificance when residential mobility into the areas is taken into account. He states (Dunham, 1965, p. 252) "the evidence pointed very clearly to the fact that the difference in rates was due to the patterns of mobility of those families that produced schizophrenia. . . . The evidence clearly pointed to the operation of certain forces within the social system that apparently selected certain families that produced schizophrenics for certain sub-communities within the city. . . ."

Thus Dunham's position on the concentration of schizophrenics in the lowest socio-economic stratum is clear. It is a function of their disease and its disabling characteristics. He goes on to state (Dunham, 1965, p. 252) "There is no basis for asserting that one social class is likely to produce more schizophrenics than another social class. . . ." On the other hand, Dunham rejects "drift" as a concept, since for him, this implies an unconscious process over which the individual exerts no control. The preferable concept is "social selection." In an earlier essay, he describes the process of social selection as follows (Dunham, 1961, p. 247):

"Certain persons because of age, sex, personality traits, intelligence, emotional instability, psychotic proneness, are selected for certain positions in occupational groups, city areas, marital status categories, institutions and the like in contrast to other positions in these structures as the social system moves through time. The process may be either active or passive as far as the person is concerned and through it one can account for significant differences in the rate of mental illness."

Thus there appears to be a shift in point of view from a social causation hypothesis advanced in Dunham's early work to a social selection hypothesis in his later work. However, in a personal communication from Professor Dunham, it was pointed out that social selection is not a true opposite of social causation. Social selection can be used to explain the distribution pattern formed by admission rates, and to provide certain notions as to where to look for those social factors that might induce some psychiatric states. Social causation might be operative even though a process of social selection places more patients in some community areas than others.

The case for an inverse correlation for over-all rates of mental disorder, and schizophrenia in particular, and socio-economic status has been demonstrated in many studies and refuted in few. Dohrenwend and Dohrenwend (1969, p. 17) list twenty-five studies of the epidemiology of mental disorder where this comparison is possible. Of these, twenty show a maximum rate of mental disorder in the lowest socio-economic stratum, four show a maximum rate in the middle socio-economic group, and one shows a maximum rate in the highest stratum. While most of these studies do not deal with the geographical distribution of mental disorder in cities, they do show a strong consensus on poverty being related to measures of mental illness. Poverty areas of large cities being generally inner city areas, the relationship between poverty and mental illness is not independent of distribution patterns of mental illness among the subcommunities of a city.

Dohrenwend and Dohrenwend (1969) review at length the issue of social causation versus social selection. While unable to refute or confirm beyond doubt either proposition, they do offer a prototypic research design to test them which is sufficiently interesting to be recounted here in detail. They state (Dohrenwend and Dohrenwend, 1969, p. 167):

> "If the rate of psychological disorder in a particular social class is a function of the strength of social pressures experienced by members of this class, we should find higher rates of disorder in the disadvantaged ethnic groups. . . . By contrast, from a genetic point of view, we would expect just the opposite. For if psychological disorder is mainly an outcome of genetic endowment then we would expect the rate in a given class to be a function of social selection processes, whereby the able tend to rise or maintain high status and the disabled drift down from high status or fail to rise out of low status. Since the downward social pressure is greater on disadvantaged ethnic groups such as Negroes and Puerto Ricans, we would expect even more of their healthier members to be kept in low status, thereby diluting the rate of disorders. In contrast, with less pressure to block them, the tendency of healthy members of more advantaged ethnic groups to rise would leave a residue of disabled persons among the lower class members of these advantaged ethnic groups, thereby inflating the rate of disorder. Thus social selection should function to give a lower rate of disorder in disadvantaged ethnic groups, than in advantaged ethnic groups, social class held constant."*

Such a study as far as we know is not yet accomplished. If technically feasible, we believe it would constitute the next big step in the constant accrual of knowledge which has characterized the research area of the ecology of mental disorder since the publication of Faris and Dunham's Chicago study.

*Reprinted by permission of John Wiley & Sons, Inc.

NOTE

The view of the city as an ecosystem stemmed from the work of Robert Park who in work dating from 1916 proceeded to develop the concept of natural areas of the city.

2. EXPERIMENTAL DESIGN AND METHODOLOGY

In 1916, Robert E. Park, then associated with the University of Chicago, laid down some of the basic premises for the study of human behavior in the urban environment (Park, 1952). In that article, Park stated that the character and organization of a city are strongly affected by the population of that area and also by the concentration and distribution of that population within the urban area. Using biological concepts, Park adapted the ecological approach to the city and thus suggested that urban study revolve around the relationship of human beings to their urban environment.

Park and Burgess (1967) discussed four social processes which relate to urban life in their classic sociology text which was first published in 1921. They discussed *competition* as interaction without social control. It is a presocial struggle for survival out of which *conflict, accommodation,* and *assimilation* occur.

Conflict is related to political order and conscious order. Whereas competition does not demand contact between individuals or groups, conflict is a contest in which contact is indispensible. Competition determines the position of an individual in the community and conflict fixes his place in society. Park and Burgess discuss accommodation in terms of the social order that is fixed and established in custom and mores. Accommodation, which is social transmittal of cultural values and norms, is thus distinguished from the biological concept of

15

adaptation, which relates to organic modifications that are transmitted biologically. Thus, accommodation can be seen as a process of adjustment which relates to the organization of social relations to prevent or reduce conflict, control competition, and maintain stability in the social order. Finally, Park and Burgess discuss assimilation as the process of interpenetration and fusion by which individuals acquire personality and cultural experiences.

The "natural areas" concept was the key to Park's view of the city (Park, 1952). He noted that a number of homogeneous social areas developed in the city where people with similar social, ethnic, and economic backgrounds were segregated. The idea of studying these natural areas of the city was picked up by Park's students and resulted in a number of studies including:

1. Nels Anderson, *The Hobo* (1923)
2. Harvey Zorbaugh, *The Gold Coast and the Slum* (1929)
3. Frederick Thrasher, *The Gang* (1927)
4. Louis Wirth, *The Ghetto* (1928).

The idea that the city of Chicago could be divided into a number of natural areas for the purpose of analysis was extended further in the 1930's by the Social Science Research Committee of the University of Chicago, in cooperation with other Chicago agencies and the United States Bureau of the Census. The city of Chicago was divided into seventy-five community areas on the basis of the following (Kitagawa and Taeuber, 1963):

1. the settlement, growth, and history of the area
2. local identification with the area
3. the local trade area
4. distribution of membership of local institutions
5. natural and artificial geographic barriers.

Sociologically, the considerations for the establishment of areas revolved around the following variables (Kitagawa and Taeuber, 1963):

1. a history of each area as a community

2. a name
3. an awareness by the residents of the area of certain common interests
4. a set of local businesses and organizations oriented to the local community.

Thus, the argument can be summarized by stating that homogeneous social and cultural groups tended to congregate in a city within definite physical boundaries.

The question arises as to whether the community area boundaries of earlier historical periods are still useful today when the populations of the areas are not demographically similar. The argument put forth by Kitagawa and Taeuber (1963) is that a redefinition of the community area boundaries every ten years would destroy the usefulness of these geographical boundaries for comparative analyses. Moreover, it should be possible to follow the movement of social groups over time, while keeping the original community area boundaries, under the assumption that homogeneous social, cultural, and economic groups will still tend to congregate in groups even if they move their physical habitat. In addition, a specific community area may have several subpopulations which would categorize the area as heterogeneous rather than homogeneous, although a given subpopulation may congregate in a subsection of a community area.

THE STUDY POPULATION

Data in the present study were collected for 10,653 Chicago residents who were admitted to forty-four public and private mental institutions and psychiatric units of general hospitals from July 1, 1960 to June 30, 1961 (13 state hospitals, 18 psychiatric units of general hospitals, and 13 private psychiatric institutions).

The study population accounted for 12,519 mental hospital admissions during the period 1960-61. Specifically, 1,384 people had more than one admission during the study period. Also, 67.8% of the study population had stays in mental hospitals prior to the study period. There were 3,431 people admitted to a psychiatric inpatient unit for the first time during 1960-61 (32.2%).

Information was provided for the individual patients on the following variables:
1. Sex
2. Race
3. Marital Status
4. Chicago community area of residence
5. Institution assigned to
6. Type of institution (private sanitarium, general hospital, state hospital)
7. Date of birth
8. Place of birth
9. Prior psychiatric history
10. Diagnosis (using standard American Psychiatric Association nomenclature).

No information is available on occupation, educational history, family composition, income, and residential stability.

DEFINITIONS

Diagnosis is the primary diagnosis made by the psychiatric facility in accordance with the standard APA psychiatric nomenclature and entered in the patient's chart during his stay. Where the same patient has been admitted more than once during the study period and the primary diagnosis has changed, the diagnosis registered in the earlier admission is used.

Patient's area of residence is based on the address given by the patient as his residence upon admission and recorded in his chart. This address is used to identify the community area of which he is a resident.

Prior psychiatric history is recorded as all previous admissions to an inpatient psychiatric facility.

First admissions refer to that group of patients who were admitted for the first time to any study facility during the study period.

Readmissions refer to that group of patients who registered a previous hospital admission to any psychiatric facility.

Unduplicated admissions refers to the number of persons admitted to forty-four psychiatric facilities during the study period. Each person is counted once regardless of how many times he is admitted during the study period. (First admissions + readmissions = unduplicated admissions.)

Total admissions is the count of all admissions to a study facility during the study period.

SPECIAL PROBLEMS IN THE STUDY OF EPIDEMIOLOGIC MENTAL DISORDER

Psychiatric diagnoses are not only inherently unreliable but are frequently casually made by hospital psychiatrists who often do not see any definite relationship between the diagnosis assigned and the clinical disposition of the patient. This is often expressed in a cynical attitude towards diagnosis and profession of a greater faith in psychodynamic formulation or in lengthy description of the patient's behavior as opposed to the affixing of a standard diagnosis. It is always problematic for the researcher to assess the level of credibility that can be assigned to such data. It is better in any epidemiologic study to have a specially trained research team on hand to make a research diagnosis on any given patient independent of the hospital diagnosis, but this is difficult in studies of large numbers of patients entering many different hospitals.

Aside from the inherent unreliability of diagnosis and

the variable attitudes toward the process of making a diagnosis by psychiatrists, it appears that the cultural background, the kind of training, the social class, and possibly the work setting of the psychiatrist affects in serious ways the choice of a diagnostic label for a given patient with a given set of presenting symptoms. For example, the diagnosis of schizophrenia is much more widely applied than the diagnosis of manic-depressive psychosis in the United States. The reverse situation obtains in Denmark (Juel-Nielsen and Stromberg, 1963). Does this really mean that there are proportionally more schizophrenics in the United States and more manic-depressive psychotics in Denmark? A simpler explanation would be that diagnostic preferences differ from country to country. This latter explanation is supported by Juel-Nielsen and Stromberg. Differences in diagnostic practices and use of diagnostic terms cross-culturally have been observed by Stengel (1960), Kramer (1961), and Lin (1967).

Another interpretive problem posed by the diagnosis is the rather uniformly reported finding that the prevalence of schizophrenia, alcoholism, and senile dementia are inversely correlated with social class. The relation between social class and manic-depressive psychosis and psychoneurosis appears to be reversed. If, as Hollingshead and Redlich (1958) suggest, the psychiatric diagnosis conferred on a patient is in part a reflection of the class distance between the conferrer and the conferree, then this alone may explain the social class—mental illness relationship rather than an allegation of a true class relatedness in an etiologic sense of these disorders.

After all is said and done, however, what choices are available to the psychiatric epidemiologist with regard to classification? He can of course simply not do studies in this area. A more general choice appears to be to ac-

cept diagnosis as defined by the standard APA nomenclature as the only generally available, if imperfect, technique for classifying patients, and interpret his data cautiously. The problem is certainly not unique to psychiatric epidemiologic investigations but exists to a greater
or lesser extent in all other medical and social problem
areas.

Another avenue of approach to the problem of classification on a grosser level is to simply accept the criterion
of admission to a mental hospital as evidence of severe
and definite disruption of social competence. One may
then make certain observations about hospitalized patients as a group as opposed to other persons not in this
category. It is our feeling that there is merit to this kind
of classification system.

The latter consideration leads to an approach to the
concepts of incidence and prevalence which are difficult
issues in their own right as applied to mental illness.
True incidence would have to be established by a total
count of all persons becoming mentally ill in a given population at risk in a given time period. The problem is that
a) we have no satisfactory definition of the disease and
b) we have no satisfactory way of establishing point of
onset. A not wholly unsatisfactory way of disposing of
these issues is to define mental illness as that which
qualifies one for admission to a mental hospital and to set
the point of onset as the time of first admission to a mental hospital. The virtue of this approach is that while we
might encounter false negatives, i.e., some mentally ill
persons never go to a hospital, we would have few false
positives, i.e., few persons admitted to mental hospitals
are not mentally ill. By setting the level of disorder as one
severe enough to qualify for hospital admission, one
avoids the rather difficult and probably unresolvable issue of whether a person who goes for outpatient treat-

ment is "mentally ill" or merely having "a problem in living." But if one were so disposed, the definition of incidence could be extended to cover all first admissions to any psychiatric facility. Then the remaining problem is to determine what constitutes a psychiatric facility (is a family service agency such a facility?) and to contend with the population of mentally ill who are never seen at any psychiatric facility, assuming there is such a group.

Studies of prevalence encounter the same problem of defining mental illness. One may handle this problem in similar fashion by invoking the concept of "treated prevalence" and counting those cases which are in treatment in a mental health facility at a given point in time (point prevalence) or during a period of time (period prevalence). A more exhaustive approach to estimating prevalence is possible through the use of household surveys so well developed by Leighton and associates (1959, 1960, 1963) and Srole and associates (1962, 1963) among others. The problem with household surveys as documented by Dohrenwend and Dohrenwend (1969) is that differing conceptions of what constitutes mental illness contribute to tremendous variablility in the estimates of prevalence made in the many studies reported. Since the possibility of a standard definition of mental illness as a general category appears to be remote, the criterion of admission to a mental hospital or possibly other psychiatric facilities does not appear to be so unattractive as an alternative.

In the present study, we give relatively little emphasis to either incidence or prevalence and attempt more cautiously to stay close to the data which reflects mental hospital utilization or what we variously refer to as psychiatric casualty rate (rate of persons admitted to hospitals for psychiatric disorder) or rate of persons extruded from the community for reason of mental illness (the same).

THE USE OF
ECOLOGICAL VERSUS
INDIVIDUAL CORRELATIONS

In succeeding chapters, a number of methodological and analytical considerations will be discussed relative to particular discussions of the data. In this chapter, it is necessary to call attention to the problems involved with the ecological correlation. W. S. Robinson (1961) distinguishes between the individual and the ecological correlation. Robinson points out that the individual correlation is a correlation in which the variables are the personal attributes of individuals. The ecological correlation, on the other hand, is a correlation in which the variables are descriptive properties of groups. He then points out that the variables in an ecological correlation are quantitative while the variables in an individual correlation are qualitative. Using an example of the relationship between illiteracy and race, he found that the ecological correlation between the two was very strong but that the individual correlation between the two was very weak. He concludes that the ecological correlation is misleading and does not show the true relationship between variables. He finally argues that ecological correlations cannot be used as a substitute for individual correlations.

In a reply to Robinson, Herbert Menzel (1961) agrees that Robinson may be right in saying that ecological correlations are used only when individual correlations are not available, but he says that ecological correlations are useful in showing over-all relationships and they should thus be interpreted in this light. Ecological correlations allow the researcher to make territorial comparisons of various social problem indicators. A high ecological correlation between two social problem indicators implies that these two indicators are functions of a common underlying cause inherent not in individuals as such, but in interindividual differences and relationships. Thus, the ecological correlation allows for an analysis at the social system level of analysis. Individual correlations cannot or should not be generalized to this level. However, both types of analysis are useful and, in this book, both types of analysis will be made.

METHODS OF ANALYSIS

In the next chapter, the analysis will begin with a study of the characteristics of the admissions. This demographic analysis will be concerned with the age, sex, race, marital status, and place of birth of the study population. The admissions will be looked at in terms of their similarity to the people in the areas from which they come.

This analysis will be followed by an ecological analysis of the data. This will involve a comparison between the various community areas of Chicago, using a number of census and housing variables and social problem indicators. Ecological correlations will be utilized. This ecological analysis will continue with a spatial comparison of admissions by diagnosis. This will be followed by an analysis of admissions by type of institution to which admitted. Finally, detailed analyses will be made of high- and low-rate admission areas. This will first be done for total unduplicated admissions and then for first admissions.

3. DEMOGRAPHIC CHARACTERISTICS OF THE STUDY POPULATION

Ecology, defined as that discipline which studies the inter-relatedness of organisms and their environment, has provided a sufficiently general rubric to encompass a terrain far broader than its original designation as a branch of biology. Economists use ecology to develop techniques for the study of variations in physical and labor-force resources relevant to distance to and from markets. They develop these techniques to study national and international labor trends. Political scientists are concerned with such things as territorial variations in the size and complexity of administrative structures. They also are interested in voting patterns in different areas. Environmentalists are concerned with the effects of man's misuse of his environment and ways to correct this misuse. And finally, sociologists use ecology as a method for the study of the dimensions of the differences between rural, suburban, and urban communities. In addition, they study a given urban community by breaking it down into subcommunities to note differences in spatial patterns of given social problems. This book fits into this latter approach because it studies ecological distributions of mental disorders in the subcommunities of one large American city.

For the social scientist, ecological analysis can occur at several different levels. First, there may be a comparative study of the several subcommunities within a larger community, accomplished through the use of ecological correlations which allow the researcher to identify subcommunities on the basis of a number of predetermined characteristics. On a social system level, this data allows the researcher to make comparisons on a community level but not to generalize to an individual level.

The social ecologist is also interested in whether certain population segments of subcommunities display characteristics similar to the population at large. For example, one may be interested in whether or not those people who become mentally ill are sociologically similar to the population of the areas from which they come. Such research may also seek information which may be helpful in the identification of groups at high risk of becoming mentally ill.

In the analysis which follows in this chapter and succeeding ones, our analysis will cover interpretations at both the social system and social psychological (individual) levels. The social system analysis will be more detailed, thus providing some comparative data with previous ecological studies of mental disorders. The present chapter is concerned with an analysis of the demographic characteristics of the Chicago people admitted to mental hospitals from July 1, 1960 to June 30, 1961.

GENERAL CHARACTERISTICS
OF THE STUDY
POPULATION

Demographically, the patient population shows some interesting differences from the Chicago population as a whole. Table 1 shows more men admitted (51.6%) than women (48.4%). This is a reversal of the sex distribution of the Chicago population as a whole which is 48.6% men

TABLE 1
Demographic Comparison of Chicago People Admitted to Mental Hospitals and Chicago Populations as a Whole

Demographic Variable	Patient Population Number	Per- centage	City of Chicago Population Number	Per- centage
Sex				
Total	10,653	100.0	3,550,404	100.0
Males	5,495	51.6	1,726,986	48.6
Females	5,158	48.4	1,823,418	51.4
Race				
Total	10,653	100.0	3,550,404	100.0
White	8,698	81.6	2,712,748	76.4
Nonwhite	1,955	18.4	837,656	23.6
Age				
Total	10,653	100.0	3,550,404	100.0
Under 25	879	8.2	1,412,277	39.7
25-44	4,187	39.3	956,920	27.0
45-64	3,994	37.5	834,632	23.5
65 & over	1,593	15.0	346,575	9.8
Marital Status				
Total	10,653	100.0	2,630,047*	100.0
Single	2,957	27.8	630,051	24.0
Married	3,945	37.1	1,572,559	59.8
Separated	1,196	11.2	86,521	3.3
Widowed	1,354	12.7	251,164	9.5
Divorced	1,068	10.0	89,752	3.4
Unknown	133	1.2	—	—
Nativity†				
Total	10,653	100.0	3,550,404	100.0
Foreign born	817	7.7	438,392	12.3
US born	5,691	53.4	3,112,012	87.7
Unknown	4,145	38.9	—	—

*Population 14 years of age and over.
†Excluding the unknown, 87.4% would be native born and 12.6% foreign born.

and 51.4% women. The nonwhite population is represented in the patient population by only. 18.4%. For the United States as a whole, trend data show that there has been a striking increase in nonwhite prevalence and incidence rates over the last forty years (Pugh and Mac-

Mahon, 1962; U. S. Department of Health, Education, and Welfare, 1965). In the city as a whole, the nonwhite population accounted for 23.6% of the total population in 1960. Approximately three-quarters of the patients fall in the age groupings between 25 and 64 years (76.8%) whereas these age groupings account for only 50.5% of the citywide population. The age group over 65 years of age is overrepresented in the patient population while the age group under 25 is underrepresented in the patient population. The underrepresentation in the under 25 age group is undoubtedly affected by the relative scarcity of child and adolescent facilities in Chicago. Single people and those who are widowed, separated, and divorced are overrepresented in the patient population (61.7%); these groups account for 40.2% of the over-all population of Chicago. With nativity, there was a problem in that place of birth was not reported for all the patient population (38.9% were not reported). If the unknown group is left out of the comparison, the foreign-born patient population approximates the percentage of foreign born in the city population.

Table 2 presents a number of age-, sex-, and race-specific rates for the patient population as a whole. For the various age groups, the age-specific rates increase as the population ages increase until age 65 when a slight decline in utilization occurs. The white population shows a significantly greater rate of utilization of mental hospitals (320.6/100,000) than the nonwhite population (233.4/100,000). The age-specific rates for the white population increase with age up to age 65 and then show a decline in the over-65 age group. The nonwhite population shows a decline in utilization of mental hospitals by the 45-64 age group. The nonwhite age-specific rate for the age group over 65 is higher (503.4) than it is for the white population (454.0).

Men show an over-all higher rate of utilization (318.2) than women (282.9). Women show an almost stable age-

TABLE 2
Age-, Sex-, and Race-Specific Rates
for Chicago People Admitted to
44 Public and Private Institutions
in Fiscal Year 1961

Sex & Race	Total	Under 25	25-44	45-64	65+
A. Patients Admitted by Age, Race, & Sex					
Total	10,653	879	4,187	3,994	1,593
White male	4,488	316	1,573	1,935	664
White female	4,210	287	1,579	1,615	729
Nonwhite male	1,007	153	524	237	93
Nonwhite female	948	123	511	207	107
Total white	8,698	603	3,152	3,550	1,393
Total nonwhite	1,955	276	1,035	444	200
Total male	5,495	469	2,097	2,172	757
Total female	5,158	410	2,090	1,822	836
B. Total Population of Chicago (1960 US Census)					
Total	3,550,404	1,412,277	956,920	834,632	346,575
White male	1,325,389	495,492	356,046	335,471	138,380
White female	1,387,359	503,322	354,820	360,750	168,467
Nonwhite male	401,597	199,663	114,989	68,738	18,207
Nonwhite female	436,059	213,800	131,065	69,673	21,521
Total white	2,712,748	998,814	710,866	696,221	306,847
Total nonwhite	837,656	413,463	246,054	138,411	39,728
Total male	1,726,986	695,155	471,035	404,209	156,587
Total female	1,823,418	717,122	485,885	430,423	189,988
C. Rate of Patients Admitted per 100,000 Population					
Total	300.1	62.2	437.5	478.5	459.6
White male	338.6	63.8	441.8	576.8	479.8
White female	303.5	57.0	445.0	447.7	432.7
Nonwhite male	250.7	76.6	455.7	344.8	510.8
Nonwhite female	217.4	57.5	389.9	297.1	497.2
Total white	320.6	60.4	443.4	509.9	454.0
Total nonwhite	233.4	66.8	420.6	320.8	503.4
Total male	318.2	67.5	445.2	537.3	483.4
Total female	282.9	57.2	430.1	423.3	440.0

specific rate for all age groupings except in the 25-years-of-age-and-under group. Men show progressively higher age-specific rates until age 65 when a decline in mental hospital utilization occurs. However, despite this decline, men still show a higher age-specific rate in the over-65 group (483.4) than women (440.0). Males, regardless of race, show a greater utilization of mental hospitals than women.

Thus far, the data has been presented for the city of Chicago as a whole. Now we will look at the same data broken down into community areas.

Sex

Table B-1 in Appendix B shows rates per 100,000 by sex for the population fifteen years of age and over. The admission rate for Chicago as a whole is still higher for males (425.8) than for females (381.4) when sex- and age-specific (adult population) rates are computed. However, it is interesting to note that women show higher utilization rates than men in more community areas in spite of greater over-all utilization by men. Women show more stable utilization patterns than men regardless of place of residence (Table 3). Men show more extremes from very low to very high depending on place of residence.

The sex data viewed spatially on Maps 1 and 2 (see Appendix A for a list and map of community areas) indicate that the male high-rate utilization areas are generally concentrated in the areas along the lakeshore and sur-

TABLE 3
Summary of Rates of Utilizations by Sex
and Number of Community areas

Rate/100,000 Adult Population	Number of Community Areas	
	Male	Female
0- 99	—	—
100-199	10	1
200-299	23	18
300-399	19	36
400-499	12	12
500-599	7	6
600 or more	4	2

Map 1—Unduplicated adult male admission rates

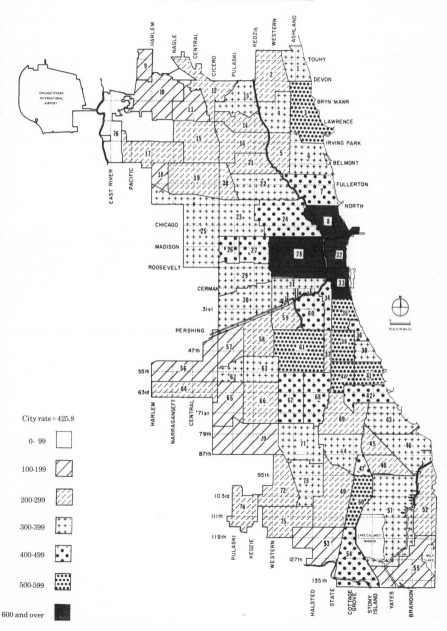

City rate = 425.8

0- 99

100-199

200-299

300-399

400-499

500-599

600 and over

Map 2—Unduplicated adult female admission rates

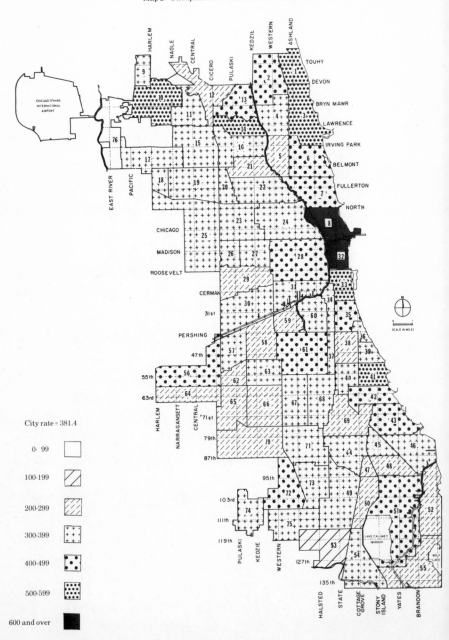

City rate = 381.4

0- 99
100-199
200-299
300-399
400-499
500-599
600 and over

rounding the Loop (C.A. 32). Another pocket of high-rate areas is in the region around Lake Calumet on the extreme southside of the city. C.A. 47 (Burnside) and C.A. 50 (Pullman) are lower-middle-class white areas. C.A. 54 (Riverdale) is primarily black. Except for these three areas, there is a very strong central spatial pattern for male admissions in Chicago. Almost all high-rate areas are contiguous, located at the city center and the lakefront.

The female pattern is less clear-cut. Although lakeshore areas and city-limit community areas generally show the highest utilization, all socio-economic levels are represented in the high-rate female areas. The males tend to be located in lower socio-economic areas on the whole.

Race

The racial data offers us the chance to investigate race in a number of ways. Table B-2 in Appendix B shows black and white hospital utilization rates using a race and adult population base. On the whole, whites utilize mental hospitals more than blacks in Chicago.

Table 4 looks at utilization rates in communities by percent of area which is black. As can be seen there is a tendency for a greater hospital use by blacks in areas which are less than ten percent black. In fact, hospital admissions were highest—about 4 per thousand—in areas which were less than five percent black. This accords with the contention that racially mixed areas are higher risk areas for mental hospitalization and further that minority status is a factor in determining extrusion from the community. When we look at white admissions relative to percent black population, white admissions show a substantial increase in areas where blacks comprise over 26 percent of the population.

TABLE 4
Utilization of Mental Hospitals
for Black and White Residents
by Percent of Community Areas
Which is Black

Percent Black	Number of Community Areas	Rate/100,000 Black Adults 15 yrs and over	Rate/100,000 White Adults 15 yrs and over
Less than 10%	51	276.0	220.0
10-25%	5	244.7	390.0
26-50%	4	232.8	580.0
51-75%	4	238.2	720.0
76-100%	11	231.4	510.0*

*The rate for whites in areas which are 90% or more Black is 550.0/100,000 White Adults 15 yrs and older.

Blacks tend to be primarily diagnosed schizophrenic regardless of sex (Table 5). White males have a large percentage (32%) of diagnosed alcoholics and schizophrenics (18%). White females are predominantly diagnosed as being either schizophrenic (28%) or psychoneurotic (29%). Women, regardless of race, tend to be diag-

TABLE 5
Breakdown of Sex and Race by Diagnosis

Diagnosis	White Males		White Females		Black Males		Black Females	
	No.	%	No.	%	No.	%	No.	%
Total	4488	100.0	4210	100.0	1001	100.0	937	100.0
Schizophrenic	802	17.9	1190	28.3	335	33.5	456	48.7
Manic-Depressive	125	2.8	331	7.9	6	0.6	15	1.6
Senile and Arterio.	449	10.0	431	10.2	100	10.0	122	13.0
Alcoholic	1444	32.2	123	2.9	124	12.4	21	2.2
PP (Psychophysiological)	4	0.1	9	0.2	3	0.3	0	0.0
PN (Psychoneurotic)	551	12.3	1231	29.2	20	2.0	63	6.7
PD (Personality Disorders)	184	4.1	201	4.8	69	6.9	40	4.3
All Others	929	20.6	694	16.5	344	34.3	220	23.5

nosed schizophrenic to a greater extent than men. Regardless of race or sex, there is approximately 10% of each group who are diagnosed senile or arteriosclerotic.

Age

As pointed out earlier in this chapter, the age distribution of people admitted to inpatient mental institutions is biased. Young people with mental problems do not end up in the statistics because of a lack of services for children and adolescents in the Chicago area. The over-65 age group is overrepresented partially due to dependency problems. Public mental hospitals have become dumping grounds for the aged without money to afford private nursing home care.

Table B-3 in Appendix B shows the age distribution of community areas in Chicago. It also shows the age distribution by community area of people admitted to mental institutions. A glance at this table shows a significant difference between the percent of the population under 24 and the percent of people admitted in this same age grouping.

Contrary to the general trend, a few areas show an underrepresentation of older admissions. These areas include Montclare (C.A. 18), Avondale (C.A. 21), Hegewisch (C.A. 55), McKinley Park (C.A. 59), Bridgeport (C.A. 60), Clearing (C.A. 64), and West Lawn (C.A. 65). These communities are predominantly white lower-middle-class communities with a large percentage (35% or more) of the population being first- or second-generation Americans. The largest group of foreign stock seems to be Poles, followed by Italians and Germans. Two other areas show an underrepresentation of people admitted over 65. The first area is the Loop (C.A. 32) which is a transient area with little residential housing. This is the central business district of Chicago and includes all the large hotels. In 1960, this area also included the skid-row section west and south of downtown. The other area is South Shore (C.A. 43). In 1960, this was primarily a Jewish area with about ten percent of the area being black. By 1970, this area had become largely black. Jews tend to use public mental hospitals little (Srole, et al., 1962). The aged Jew tends to be placed in a private home or institution if care is needed rather than in an institution labelled as a public mental hospiptal. It would appear clearly that public mental hospital admissions among the aged is related to poverty.

Marital Status

Table B-4 in Appendix B presents a percentage distribution of people admitted to public and private mental hospitals by community areas. As can be seen, the percentage of married people by community area ranges from 5 percent to 77 percent. However, in every community area except Ashburn (C.A. 70), the percent of admissions who are married is much less than the percent of married people in the population of the community area as a whole. Thus, marriage appears to give some protection to the individual as regards extrusion from the community into a mental hospital.

Table B-4 also shows a higher utilization of hospitals by people who have never married than by people who have been widowed, divorced, or separated.

This might be partially explained by the fact that mentally ill people may never marry because of their difficulty in relating in a satisfactory and stable way to others. The issue of whether admissions of single persons is higher because of their failure to marry (due to emotional problems) or whether marriage is a protection against extrusion into a mental hospital is not resolvable from the type of data presented here.

Place of Birth

Table B-5 in Appendix B shows that most people who were admitted show the United States as their place of birth. This is a consistent finding in every community area. However, the foreign-born admissions do run high in some areas. For example, West Town (C.A. 24) shows 24.5% of its people admitted as being foreign born. West Town has a large Polish population, followed by Russians, Italians, and Germans. In fact, half of the community area is made up of first- and second-generation people. Other high percentage foreign-born admission areas also show large numbers of foreign stock in the area.

CONCLUSIONS

In this chapter, we have tried to give an overview of our study by concentrating our analysis on the demographic characteristics of people admitted during the study period. It is unfortunate that our analysis lacked data on last occupation of people admitted, education, and religion.

Some of the major findings of the analysis are:

(1) More Chicago men were admitted to mental institutions than women for the city as a whole, a reversal of the sex distribution in the Chicago population.

(2) Women show more stable utilization patterns than men regardless of place of residence.

(3) Male admissions tend to be located in lower socio-economic areas on the whole while female admissions seem to come from areas of all socio-economic levels.

(4) Eighteen percent of the people admitted were non-white, a figure below the projection in the city population. Specifically, blacks utilize mental hospitals much

less than their percentage in the population would indicate they should.

(5) Black admissions are highest in those areas with the smallest percentage of black residents.

(6) Blacks are primarily diagnosed schizophrenic regardless of sex.

(7) White males have a very large percentage of diagnosed alcoholics.

(8) White females are diagnosed predominantly as either schizophrenic or psychoneurotic.

(9) Women, regardless of race, tend to be diagnosed schizophrenic to a greater extent than men.

(10) Younger people under 25 years of age are underrepresented in the patient population in comparison to their representation in the Chicago population at large and people over 65 are overrepresented.

(11) Those community areas which show an underrepresentation of geriatric admissions were generally white lower-middle-class communities with a large percentage of foreign stock.

(12) The patient population showed proportionately more single, widowed, separated, and divorced people than in the population at large.

(13) Married people utilize mental hospitals less than people who are not married.

(14) There is a higher utilization of hospitals by people who have never married than by people who have been widowed, divorced, or separated.

(15) Most admissions were born in the United States. Both the American-born and the foreign-born patient population approximate their respective percentages in the city population.

4. ECOLOGICAL ANALYSIS OF MENTAL DISORDER IN CHICAGO

The previous chapter was concerned with the individual characteristics of users of public and private mental institutions. This chapter is concerned with characteristics of Chicago communities and the relationship of these characteristics to mental hospital utilization by city residents. Herbert Menzel has argued (1961) that ecological correlations show the relationship among various social problem indicators, which help the investigator in his search for the underlying cause inherent not in the individual as such, but rather in the community relationships in which these individuals are involved. Thus, both the individual and ecological correlations are important as long as the investigator realizes the different types of information which are gotten from each type of analysis.

ECOLOGICAL CORRELATIONS

In order to determine community profiles, an intercorrelation matrix of 34 variables was computed. As can be seen in Tables 6 and 7, a large number of the variables used are based on the mental hospital utilization rates collected in the present study. These variables include information on unduplicated admissions by diagnosis, first admissions for all diagnoses and for schizophrenia, and unduplicated readmissions by diagnosis. As men-

39

TABLE 6
Variables Used in the Ecological Correlation Matrix and Factor Analysis of Characteristics Describing the 74 Community Areas

Variable No.	Description
	Mental Health
1.	Unduplicated admissions for all diagnoses (rate/100,000 population)
2.	Unduplicated schizophrenics (rate/100,000 population 15-64)
3.	Unduplicated manic-depressives (rate/100,000 population 15 and over)
4.	Unduplicated senile & arteriosclerotics (rate/100,000 population 65 and over)
5.	Unduplicated alcoholics (rate/100,000 population 15 and over)
6.	Unduplicated PP, PN, & PD (rate/100,000 population 15 and over)
7.	First admission schizophrenics (rate/100,000 population 15-64)
8.	Readmission schizophrenics (rate/100,000 population 15-64)
9.	Readmission manic-depressives (rate/100,000 population 15 and over)
10.	Readmission senile & arteriosclerotics (rate/100,000 population 65 and over)
11.	Readmission alcoholics (rate/100,000 population 15 and over)
12.	Readmission PP, PN, &PD (rate/100,000 population 15 and over)
13.	First admissions—44 mental hospitals (total)(rate/100,000 population)
14.	First admissions—State hospitals (rate/100,000 population)
15.	First admissions—Psych units of general hospitals (rate/100,000 population)
16.	First admissions—Private mental hospitals (rate/100,000 population)
17.	Admissions to state facilities for 1967 (rate/100,000 population)
	Social problems
18.	% in substandard housing [a]
19.	% illegitimate births [b]
20.	% on public assistance (1962) [b]
21.	% unemployed [a]
22.	Male delinquency rate [b]
23.	Average suicide rate [c]

TABLE 6 (Continued)

Variables Used in the Ecological Correlation Matrix and Factor Analysis of Characteristics Describing the 74 Community Areas

Variable No.	Description
	Demography
24.	Population per household [a]
25.	% Black [a]
26.	% foreign born [a]
27.	% foreign stock [a]
28.	% of population 18 years old or younger [a]
29.	% of population 65 years old or older [a]
30.	% of population with income of $3,000 or less per year [a]
31.	% of population with income of $10,000 or more per year [a]
32.	% male white-collar workers [a]
33.	% of 1960 residents now in different housing [a]
34.	Median school years completed [a]

[a] Kitagawa, E. M., and Taueber, K. E. (Eds.) *Local community fact book: Chicago metropolitan area, 1960.* Chicago: University of Chicago, 1963.
[b] Chicago, Welfare Council of, *Chicago community area profiles.* Chicago: Research dept., Welfare Council of Metropolitan Chicago., Pub. No. 4006, 1964.
[c] Maris, R. *Social forces in urban suicide.* Homewood, Ill.: Dorsey Press, 1969.

41

TABLE 7
Ecological Correlation Matrix for 34 Variables

Description	1	2	3	4	5	6	7	8
Mental Health								
1. Unduplicated admissions (all diag.)	1.0000							
2. Unduplicated schizophrenics	0.6439	1.0000						
3. Unduplicated manic-depressives	0.1048	-0.2022	1.0000					
4. Unduplicated Senile & arteriosclerotics	0.4605	0.5633	-0.3756	1.0000				
5. Unduplicated alcoholics	0.8139	0.5309	-0.1773	0.5786	1.0000			
6. Unduplicated PP, PN, & PD	0.3343	-0.1024	0.6200	-0.2736	-0.0289	1.0000		
7. First admission schizophrenics	0.0691	0.0788	0.1172	-0.1972	-0.0534	0.2474	1.0000	
8. Readmission schizophrenics	0.5990	0.9397	-0.2357	0.6119	0.5330	-0.1836	-0.2669	1.0000
9. Readmission manic-depressives	0.1841	-0.0953	0.8169	-0.2777	-0.0883	0.4374	0.1015	-0.1274
10. Readmission senile & arteriosclerotics	0.4512	0.5550	-0.3409	0.9581	0.5780	-0.2650	-0.3263	0.6484
11. Readmission alcoholics	0.7917	0.5528	-0.2172	0.6255	0.9867	-0.0866	-0.0844	0.5634
12. Readmission PP, PN, & PD	0.5474	0.2206	0.4798	-0.0486	0.1942	0.7676	0.0685	0.1896
13. First admissions—44 mental hospitals	0.5465	-0.0622	0.4879	-0.1671	0.2755	0.7814	0.4566	-0.2164
14. First admissions—State hospitals	0.8041	0.5136	-0.0756	0.4715	0.9168	0.0346	-0.0583	0.5164
15. First admissions—Psych. units	0.1722	-0.2691	0.5260	-0.3523	-0.1642	0.7964	0.4671	-0.4197
16. First admissions—Private hospitals	0.0086	-0.3423	0.3837	-0.4015	-0.2209	0.5000	0.3839	-0.4627
17. Admissions to state fac. for 1967	0.7215	0.6921	-0.2172	0.6728	0.7651	-0.2204	-0.2830	0.7663
Social Problems								
18. % in substandard housing	0.5707	0.7088	-0.4314	0.6998	0.6257	-0.2751	-0.2234	0.7610
19. % illegitimate births	0.3453	0.6222	-0.4244	0.6319	0.3950	-0.2816	-0.3193	0.7112
20. % on public assistance (1962)	0.2968	0.7163	-0.4177	0.7333	0.4071	-0.3747	-0.3273	0.8047
21. % unemployed	0.2911	0.7103	-0.3964	0.7050	0.4083	-0.4060	-0.3205	0.7962
22. Male delinquency rate	0.4648	0.7547	-0.4488	0.7120	0.5315	-0.3641	-0.2492	0.8147
23. Average suicide rate	0.5437	0.0953	0.1387	-0.1175	0.3321	0.3938	0.0632	0.0705

TABLE 7 (Continued)
Ecological Correlation Matrix for 34 Variables

Description	1	2	3	4	5	6	7	8
Demography								
24. Population per household	-0.5430	-0.1081	-0.1934	0.1363	-0.1791	-0.3844	-0.1958	-0.0375
25. % Black	0.1859	0.6032	-0.4058	0.6690	0.2679	-0.4303	-0.3808	0.7138
26. % foreign born	0.0321	-0.2840	0.3474	-0.5632	-0.1638	0.3522	0.2687	-0.3668
27. % foreign stock	-0.1894	-0.5465	0.3950	-0.7050	-0.3124	0.3893	0.3228	-0.6394
28. % of population ≦ 18	-0.2205	0.3003	-0.3601	0.4598	0.1176	-0.3918	-0.2396	0.3723
29. % of population ≧ 65	0.2448	-0.2434	0.4315	-0.4502	-0.1240	0.4922	0.2668	-0.3266
30. % of population with income ≦ $3,000	0.4111	0.7732	-0.3935	0.7227	0.4898	-0.3203	-0.2958	0.8488
31. % of population with income ≧ $10,000	-0.2355	-0.6621	0.4267	-0.4800	-0.3762	0.5333	0.2607	-0.7292
32. % male white collar workers	0.1292	-0.3503	0.5144	-0.3219	-0.1924	0.7488	0.2027	-0.4077
33. % 1960 residents in diff. house	0.4209	0.6030	-0.1601	0.5288	0.3677	-0.1143	-0.1606	0.6385
34. Median school year completed	0.0007	-0.3130	0.4556	-0.2326	-0.2550	0.6158	0.1566	-0.3553

TABLE 7 (Continued)
Ecological Correlation Matrix for 34 Variables

	Description	9	10	11	12	13	14	15	16
	Mental Health								
1.	Unduplicated admissions (all diag.)								
2.	Unduplicated schizophrenics								
3.	Unduplicated manic-depressives								
4.	Unduplicated senile & arteriosclerotics								
5.	Unduplicated alcoholics								
6.	Unduplicated PP, PN, & PD								
7.	First admission schizophrenics								
8.	Readmission schizophrenics								
9.	Readmission manic-depressives	1.0000							
10.	Readmission senile & arteriosclerotics	-0.2490	1.0000						
11.	Readmission alcoholics	-0.1134	0.6181	1.0000					
12.	Readmission PP, PN, & PD	0.3772	0.0117	0.1436	1.0000				
13.	First admissions—44 mental hospitals	0.3815	-0.2342	0.2001	0.5388	1.0000			
14.	First admissions—State hospitals	-0.0048	0.4775	0.8688	0.2632	0.3468	1.0000		
15.	First admissions—Psych. units	0.3678	-0.4248	-0.2010	0.4724	0.7894	-0.1526	1.0000	
16.	First admissions—Private hospitals	0.3029	-0.4488	-0.2779	0.1751	0.6334	-0.1765	0.4246	1.0000
17.	Admissions to state fac. for 1967	-0.0992	0.7138	0.7949	0.1355	-0.0802	0.7156	-0.4064	-0.4129
	Social Problems								
18.	% in substandard housing	-0.2616	0.7244	0.6488	0.1040	-0.2011	0.5713	-0.4880	-0.3870
19.	% illegitimate births	-0.3316	0.6550	0.4574	0.0667	-0.3695	0.3235	-0.4372	-0.5527
20.	% on public assistance (1962)	-0.3722	0.7531	0.4618	0.0025	-0.4527	0.3401	-0.5729	-0.5507
21.	% unemployed	-0.3097	0.7486	0.4600	-0.0181	-0.4838	0.3579	-0.6415	-0.5358
22.	Male delinquency rate	-0.2913	0.7345	0.5794	0.0154	-0.3429	0.4722	-0.5550	-0.4872
23.	Average suicide rate	0.1200	-0.1193	0.2753	0.4185	0.5482	0.3762	0.2945	0.3393

44

TABLE 7 (Continued)
Ecological Correlation Matrix for 34 Variables

	Description	9	10	11	12	13	14	15	16
	Demography								
24.	Population per household	-0.2640	0.1509	-0.1566	-0.4517	0.5413	-0.2145	-0.3746	0.3932
25.	% Black	-0.3331	0.7082	0.3418	-0.0937	-0.5528	0.2012	-0.5669	-0.6216
26.	% foreign born	0.3707	-0.5921	-0.2106	0.1658	0.4662	-0.0881	0.3837	0.5740
27.	% foreign stock	0.3685	-0.7356	-0.3735	0.0847	0.4869	-0.2430	0.4965	0.6319
28.	% of population ≦ 18	-0.4075	0.4763	0.1411	-0.2744	-0.5476	0.0645	-0.5321	-0.4981
29.	% of population ≧ 65	0.4040	-0.4838	-0.1677	0.3817	0.6216	-0.0462	0.5687	0.5867
30.	% of population with income ≦ $3,000	-0.3273	0.7480	0.5344	0.0690	-0.3590	0.4251	-0.5510	-0.4732
31.	% of population with income ≧ $10,000	0.2708	-0.5280	-0.4192	0.2126	0.4993	-0.3329	0.7204	0.4167
32.	% male white collar workers	0.3317	-0.3624	-0.2244	0.4929	0.6661	-0.1581	0.8253	0.4228
33.	% 1960 residents in diff. house	-0.1030	0.5478	0.4195	0.1392	-0.1585	0.3102	-0.2323	-0.3745
34.	Median school year completed	0.2306	-0.2637	-0.2797	0.3521	0.4760	-0.2169	0.7128	0.2345

45

TABLE 7 (Continued)
Ecological Correlation Matrix for 34 Variables

Description	17	18	19	20	21	22	23	24
Mental Health								
1. Unduplicated admissions (all diag.)								
2. Unduplicated schizophrenics								
3. Unduplicated manic-depressives								
4. Unduplicated senile & arteriosclerotics								
5. Unduplicated alcoholics								
6. Unduplicated PP, PN, & PD								
7. First admission schizophrenics								
8. Readmission schizophrenics								
9. Readmission manic-depressives								
10. Readmission senile & arteriosclerotics								
11. Readmission alcoholics								
12. Readmission PP, PN, & PD								
13. First admissions—44 mental hospitals								
14. First admissions—State hospitals								
15. First admissions—Psych. units								
16. First admissions—Private hospitals								
17. Admissions to state fac. for 1967	1.0000							
Social Problems								
18. % in substandard housing	0.7791	1.0000						
19. % illegitimate births	0.6703	0.6856	1.0000					
20. % on public assistance (1962)	0.6810	0.7304	0.8489	1.0000				
21. % unemployed	0.7001	0.7507	0.8050	0.9417	1.0000			
22. Male delinquency rate	0.7968	0.8676	0.8414	0.8660	0.8604	1.0000		
23. Average suicide rate	0.1666	0.2027	-0.1430	-0.2477	-0.2537	0.0133	1.0000	

TABLE 7 (Continued)
Ecological Correlation Matrix for 34 Variables

	Description	17	18	19	20	21	22	23	24
	Demography								
24.	Population per household	-0.2130	-0.1804	0.0824	0.2513	0.2397	-0.0186	-0.6828	1.0000
25.	% Black	0.6534	0.6209	0.8456	0.8900	0.8961	0.8373	-0.3359	0.2357
26.	% foreign born	-0.3778	-0.3817	-0.5780	-0.6659	-0.6405	-0.5845	0.4409	-0.4084
27.	% foreign stock	-0.6377	-0.6058	-0.7760	-0.8496	-0.8364	-0.8159	0.2879	-0.2620
28.	% of population ≦ 18	0.1271	0.2711	0.4023	0.6339	0.6110	0.3838	-0.5107	0.83/7
29.	% of population ≧ 65	-0.1588	-0.2968	-0.4468	-0.5582	-0.5510	-0.4261	0.4775	0.7287
30.	% of population with income ≦ $3,000	0.7240	0.7849	0.8115	0.9610	0.9553	0.8630	-0.1312	0.1423
31.	% of population with income ≧ $10,000	-0.6337	-0.6731	-0.5556	-0.6823	-0.7703	-0.7351	0.0830	-0.1125
32.	% male white collar workers	-0.3469	-0.4603	-0.3112	-0.4741	-0.5652	-0.5005	0.2928	-0.3813
33.	% 1960 residents in diff. house	0.6407	0.4926	0.6305	0.6274	0.5767	0.7158	0.0990	-0.1228
34.	Median school year completed	-0.3245	-0.4791	-0.2575	-0.3654	-0.4645	-0.4353	0.1284	-0.1812

TABLE 7 (Continued)
Ecological Correlation Matrix for 34 Variables

Description	25	26	27	28	29	30	31	32
Mental Health								
1. Unduplicated admissions (all diag.)								
2. Unduplicated schizophrenics								
3. Unduplicated manic-depressives								
4. Unduplicated senile & arteriosclerotics								
5. Unduplicated alcoholics								
6. Unduplicated PP, PN, & PD								
7. First admission schizophrenics								
8. Readmission schizophrenics								
9. Readmission manic-depressives								
10. Readmission senile & arteriosclerotics								
11. Readmission alcoholics								
12. Readmission PP, PN, & PD								
13. First admissions—44 mental hospitals								
14. First admissions—State hospitals								
15. First admissions—Psych. units								
16. First admissions—Private hospitals								
17. Admissions to state fac. for 1967								
Social Problems								
18. % in substandard housing								
19. % illegitimate births								
20. % on public assistance (1962)								
21. % unemployed								
22. Male delinquency rate								
23. Average suicide rate								

48

TABLE 7 (Continued)
Ecological Correlation Matrix for 34 Variables

Description	25	26	27	28	29	30	31	32
Demography								
24. Population per household								
25. % Black	1.0000							
26. % foreign born	-0.7783	1.0000						
27. % foreign stock	-0.9373	0.9062	1.0000					
28. % of population $\leq$ 18	0.4957	-0.5661	-0.5418	1.0000				
29. % of population $\geq$ 65	-0.5297	0.6197	0.5737	-0.8577	1.0000			
30. % of population with income $\leq$ $3,000	0.8381	-0.5550	-0.7798	0.5692	-0.4442	1.0000		
31. % of population with income $\geq$ $10,000	-0.6121	0.2488	0.5126	-0.4275	0.4115	-0.7362	1.0000	
32. % male white collar workers	-0.4109	0.2497	0.3606	-0.5186	0.5404	-0.4758	0.8366	1.0000
33. % 1960 residents in diff. house	0.6601	-0.4199	-0.6548	0.1905	-0.3511	0.5757	-0.5054	-0.1754
34. Median school year completed	-0.2435	-0.0256	0.1277	-0.3190	0.2880	-0.4292	0.7837	0.8818

TABLE 7 (Continued)
Ecological Correlation Matrix for 34 Variables

Description	33	34
Mental Health		
1. Unduplicated admissions (all diag.)		
2. Unduplicated schizophrenics		
3. Unduplicated manic-depressives		
4. Unduplicated senile & arteriosclerotics		
5. Unduplicated alcoholics		
6. Unduplicated PP, PN, & PD		
7. First admission schizophrenics		
8. Readmission schizophrenics		
9. Readmission manic-depressives		
10. Readmission senile & arteriosclerotics		
11. Readmission alcoholics		
12. Readmission PP, PN, & PD		
13. First admissions—44 mental hospitals		
14. First admissions—State hospitals		
15. First admissions—Psych. units		
16. First admissions—Private hospitals		
17. Admissions to state fac. for 1967		
Social Problems		
18. % in substandard housing		
19. % illegitimate births		
20. % on public assistance (1962)		
21. % unemployed		
22. Male delinquency rate		
23. Average suicide rate		

TABLE 7 (Continued)
Ecological Correlation Matrix for 34 Variables

Description	33	34
Demography		
24. Population per household		
25. % Black		
26. % foreign born		
27. % foreign stock		
28. % of population $\leq$ 18		
29. % of population $\geq$ 65		
30. % of population with income $\leq$ $3,000		
31. % of population with income $\geq$ $10,000		
32. % male white collar workers		
33. % 1960 residents in diff. house	1.0000	
34. Median school year completed	-0.0373	1.0000

tioned earlier, first admissions plus unduplicated readmissions add up to total unduplicated admissions. The
correlations include a number of social problem indicators and standard census variables.

It was decided to compute the ecological correlations
on the basis of 74 community areas excluding the Loop
(C.A. 32) or central business district, because the small
population base and its over-all transient character affects the correlations greatly. There are a number of hotels which have some permanent residents of higher income groups but which mostly serve transient populations. Of the Loop population, 41.6% had incomes over
$10,000 a year in 1960. However, resident use in the area
is primarily limited to housing in the slum and skid-row
areas, whose residents, incidentally, are very likely un-
derenumerated in the U. S. Census. A demonstration of
how the Loop affects the ecological correlations can be
seen in the following examples: The ecological correlation between unduplicated schizophrenic admissions
and percent of community area with an income under
$3000 was 0.77 without the Loop and 0.35 with the Loop
included. Another example is the ecological correlation
between unduplicated schizophrenic admissions and percent of community area with income over $10,000 where
the correlation was -0.12 with the Loop and -0.66 without
the Loop included.

MAJOR FINDINGS

Total Unduplicated Admissions

The major finding with respect to persons admitted to
hospitals with a psychiatric diagnosis during the study
period from Chicago is that the people who demonstrate
the highest utilization of mental institutions tend to
come from areas with high percentages of poor people (r =

0.41) and high percentages of substandard housing (0.57). The high mental hospital utilization areas also tend to be areas which lack residential stability (0.42). The areas also tend to be high delinquency areas (0.46) and areas with high rates of successful suicides (0.54).

It is worthwhile in passing to note that state hospital admission rates in 1967 correlate highly (0.72) with the unduplicated admission rate in 1961. This would seem to indicate that high utilization areas during the study period remained high six years after the study was completed.

Total First Admissions

With regard to first admissions as a whole, some interesting variations in pattern are found which contrast sharply with the findings on unduplicated admissions. First admissions tend to come from areas with more economically affluent populations (0.50), with higher median education (0.48), and a larger percentage of white-collar employees (0.67). First admissions also tend to use private sanitaria (0.63) and psychiatric units of general hospitals (0.79) rather than state hospitals (0.35).

Schizophrenia

Many of Faris and Dunham's findings relate to first admission schizophrenia. Very weak relationships were found between the income variables: income under $3000, r = -0.30; income over $10,000, r = 0.26, which implies that first admission schizophrenics can come from any area of the city. However, with the total unduplicated schizophrenic admissions, the correlations related to income become stronger. Schizophrenics come from areas with poor populations (0.77) and large percentages of substandard housing (0.71). The high utilization areas also correlate highly with the residential mobility variable (0.60) and with high unemployment (0.71). Schizophrenics also tend to come from areas with high male delinquency rates (0.75), percent illegitimate births (0.62), and percent public assistance recipients (0.72). Another interesting finding relates to unduplicated readmissions. A correlation of 0.85 was found between readmitted schizophrenics and income under $3,000, whereas the correlation between readmitted schizophrenics and income over $10,000 is -0.73.

Manic-Depressive Psychosis

The manic-depressive diagnostic group does not tend to come from areas with a large percentage of blacks (-0.41) but does tend to come from areas with a larger percentage of foreign stock (0.40). Manic-depressive patients tend to come from economically more affluent areas (0.43) with higher median school years completed (0.46). The areas also tend to have large percentages of white-collar employees (0.51). Male delinquency tends to be lower in the areas from which this diagnostic group comes (-0.45).

Diseases of the Senium

Those people diagnosed as senile and/or arteriosclerotic tend to come from areas with large black populations (0.67), small aged populations (-0.45), and tend to have smaller foreign-born populations (-0.56). These patients also come from relatively poorer areas of the city (0.72) with large percentages of substandard housing (0.70). The neighborhoods tend to be characterized by residential mobility (0.53) with high unemployment rates (0.71). The delinquency rate also tends to be high in the areas from which these people come (0.71), as are the rates on percentage of illegitimate births (0.63) and percentage on public assistance (0.73).

Alcoholism

Alcoholic patients tend to come from low-income areas (0.49) with high percentages of substandard housing (0.63). There is a tendency, although weak, for these patients to come from high unemployment areas (0.41) and also areas with some transiency (0.37). These areas of alcoholic admissions also tend to be high on male delinquency (0.53), the percentage of illegitimate births (0.40), and the percentage on public assistance (0.41). The ecological relationships are on the whole much more difficult to evaluate for the alcoholic group. Not all alcoholics go to mental hospitals. Many go to jail. Further research is needed into the factors which lead the alcoholic into a mental institution rather than a jail.

Psychophysiological, Psychoneurotic, and Personality Disorders

The strongest relationship found for the psychophysiological, psychoneurotic, and personality disorders diagnostic groups is that they tend to come from high-income areas (0.53) with higher median school years completed (0.62) and a high percentage of white-collar employees (0.75). There is also a tendency for these areas to have a small black population (-0.43). Considering the fact that the data in this study exclude outpatient facilities and private psychiatrists, the findings for these diagnoses present some interesting hypotheses as to whether there is a relationship between social class and the diagnoses of psychophysiological, psychoneurotic, and personality disorders similar to the findings reported by Hollingshead and Redlich (1958). Unfortunately, the data in this study do not allow us to directly test these hypotheses since no information is available on the patient population with respect to occupation, education, and income.

TABLE 8
Factor Loadings of the 34 Variables used in the Analysis of the 74 Community Areas

Variables	1	2	3	4	5	6	7	8
Mental Health								
1. Unduplicated admissions (all diag.)	0.3783	0.3662	-0.1558	0.7696	0.1579	-0.1158	0.2066	0.0442
2. Unduplicated schizophrenics	0.7324	0.0110	0.2250	0.3504	0.0586	-0.3330	0.3050	-0.1042
3. Unduplicated manic-depressives	-0.2427	0.0893	-0.3715	-0.0497	0.8269	0.0083	0.1427	0.0379
4. Unduplicated senile & arterio.	0.6743	-0.2241	0.0579	0.4662	-0.1347	0.0315	-0.2571	0.2666
5. Unduplicated alcoholics	0.2605	0.0192	0.0724	0.9452	-0.0533	-0.0077	0.0134	-0.0181
6. Unduplicated PP, PN, & PD	-0.1594	0.2018	-0.7074	0.0752	0.2955	-0.0935	0.4627	0.1969
7. First admission schizophrenics	-0.2132	0.1027	-0.1529	-0.0039	-0.0089	-0.9260	-0.0141	0.0623
8. Readmission schizophrenics	0.7812	-0.0246	0.2692	0.3401	0.0594	-0.0043	0.2995	-0.1229
9. Readmission manic-depressives	-0.1837	0.1916	-0.1338	0.0197	0.9078	-0.0185	0.0168	0.0089
10. Readmission senile & arterio.	0.6979	-0.2348	0.0896	0.4536	-0.0791	0.1674	-0.2041	0.2374
11. Readmission alcoholics	0.3224	0.0111	0.0966	0.9095	-0.0612	-0.0039	-0.0389	-0.0401
12. Readmission PP, PN, & PD	0.1855	0.2534	-0.5053	0.1864	0.3142	0.0540	0.5848	0.0864
13. First admissions—44 mental hosp.	-0.3136	0.3629	-0.5594	0.4272	0.1863	-0.3100	0.1988	0.2465
14. First admissions—State hosp.	0.2047	0.0524	0.0678	0.9153	0.0275	0.0411	0.1016	-0.0398
15. First admissions—Psych units	-0.3383	0.2362	-0.7570	-0.0106	0.1666	-0.3112	0.1363	0.0244
16. First admissions—Private hosp.	-0.4366	0.3978	-0.1758	-0.1123	0.1319	-0.2393	0.1196	0.5753
17. Admissions to state facilities for 1967	0.6674	0.1662	0.2154	0.6066	0.0567	0.1293	-0.0876	-0.0985
Social Problems								
18. % in substandard housing	0.6791	0.1218	0.3256	0.4535	-0.1938	0.0890	0.1008	0.1001
19. % illegitimate births	0.8358	-0.0890	0.0980	0.1517	-0.1918	0.1329	0.0358	-0.1026
20. % on public assistance in 1962	0.8719	-0.2794	0.2240	0.1594	-0.1368	0.0850	0.0725	0.0406
21. % unemployed	0.8480	-0.2586	0.3393	0.1633	-0.0609	0.0863	0.0565	0.0706
22. Male delinquency rates	0.8520	0.0145	0.2939	0.2943	-0.1472	0.0329	-0.0024	-0.0622
23. Average suicide rates	-0.1459	0.6461	-0.1506	0.4036	-0.1159	0.0733	0.3787	-0.0630

TABLE 8 (Continued)
Factor Loadings of the 34 Variables used in the Analysis of the 74 Community Areas

Variables	1	2	3	4	5	6	7	8
Demography								
24. Population per household	-0.0338	-0.9318	0.1663	-0.1741	-0.0655	0.0796	-0.0789	-0.0231
25. % Black	0.9041	-0.2004	0.1560	0.0095	-0.0971	0.1496	-0.1662	-0.1054
26. % foreign born	-0.6633	0.4430	0.1270	0.0110	0.1911	-0.1335	0.3708	0.0922
27. % foreign stock	-0.8661	0.2719	-0.0237	-0.0856	0.1556	-0.1276	0.2409	0.1260
28. % of population ≦ 18 years old	0.3361	-0.8640	0.2293	0.0257	-0.1797	0.0494	0.1234	0.0455
29. % of population ≧ 65 years old	-0.3343	0.7614	-0.2309	-0.0348	0.2230	-0.0752	0.0708	0.1976
30. % of population with ≦ $3,000 income	0.8456	-0.1841	0.2790	0.2446	-0.1100	0.0635	0.1611	0.1187
31. % of population with ≧ $10,000 income	-0.5491	0.0477	-0.7467	-0.1877	0.0364	0.0065	-0.1320	0.0602
32. % male white collar workers	-0.2245	0.2698	-0.8837	-0.0797	0.1213	0.0028	0.0545	0.0501
33. % of 1960 residents in diff. house	0.7456	0.0840	-0.0176	0.1858	0.0275	-0.0499	-0.0199	-0.3573
34. Median school year completed	-0.1077	0.0662	-0.9219	-0.1590	0.0938	-0.0052	-0.0857	-0.1132

57

FACTOR ANALYSIS

The demographic and social data presented above was further analyzed utilizing Factor Analysis (Principal Component Solution). It was felt that this further analysis would allow us to determine the presence of one or more underlying factors which are related (in varying degrees) to the social indices utilized in this study.

Table 8 shows the factor loadings of the thirty-four variables used in the analysis of the seventy-four community areas after rotation. The eight factors shown account for 90 percent of the variance. Specifically, factor I accounts for 45 percent of the total variance; factor II for 20 percent of the variance; factor III for 8 percent of the variance; and the remaining four factors account for 17 percent of the variance. Thus the first three factors alone account for over seventy percent of the variance.

Factor I largely represents an underlying poverty factor since the highest loadings are for variables which are usually associated with poverty. The variables with high loadings (0.50 or over) include percent black, percentage with low income (less than $3000 a year), substandard housing, residential mobility, unemployment, and number of people on public assistance. This factor is high on male delinquency rates, illegitimacy, schizophrenic hospital admissions for 1960-1961, senile and arteriosclerotic admissions for 1960-1961, and admission rates to state hospitals in 1967-1968. One interesting negative loading is percent foreign born.

Factor II appears to be an isolation factor. Mental hospital variables show low loadings on this factor. The variables with high positive loadings for this factor include suicides and percent of population over 65 years of age. The variables with high negative loadings include population per household and percent of the population 18 years of age and younger. Although the loading is not as high as other variables, this factor shows a tendency for the areas to have large foreign-born populations. What we seem to find in this factor are communities where people are alone and with very few interactional ties.

Factor III, which shows high negative loadings, appears to represent an upper-middle-class socio-economic factor. Thus factor III seems to be the obverse of factor I. The high negative loadings include percent of the community with incomes over $10,000 a year, median school years completed, and percent of white-collar workers. This factor also shows high loadings on first admissions specifically to psychiatric wards of general hospitals. There is also a high loading for the admissions with a psychophysiological, psychoneurotic, or personality disorder diagnosis.

This analysis shows some rather interesting community profiles. It supports the argument that poverty areas not only have economic problems with which to contend but also a larger number of social problems. This analysis also gives support to the argument that people from middle-class communities tend to be labelled with less severe diagnoses when psychiatric hospitalization is needed. Finally, the isolation factor presents some interesting possibilities for research. For example, to what extent is suicide an alternative to mental hospital or nursing home utilization?

DISCUSSION

The Evidence for a Drift or Social Selection Hypothesis

First admissions for all diagnoses are recorded as higher from areas which may mainly be described as white, nonpoverty areas of the city. These first admissions appear to be routed most frequently to psychiatric units of general hospitals and private psychiatric hospitals. This finding may be contrasted with the observation that unduplicated admissions most frequently originate in areas associated with poverty and social disorganization. The following explanation, while certainly not obligatory, is consonant with the data.

The person having a first episode of severe mental disorder who lives in a well-structured, middle-class community and is in all probability covered by hospitalization insurance will seek treatment in a private rather than a public facility. Chances are that his treatment will be more effective and recovery take place in a relatively briefer period of time than in an overcrowded and understaffed state mental hospital. Also, the prospect of entering a private facility is so much more agreeable than that of entering a state hospital that one may assume persons will seek aid earlier and more willingly, thus again improving their chances for stable recovery. Upon discharge the patient's chances of avoiding subsequent readmission are held to be much better if his first admission originated in a middle-class area.

Following release from initial hospitalization, it is possible that those patients most devastated by the episode of mental illness and thus the best candidates for subsequent readmissions may actually drift to (or select)[1] other areas of the city to which they will move. These areas will presumably be less socially demanding and more in line with his impaired earning ability.

If the above process in fact occurs, then one has an explanation for the higher first admission rates (with no subsequent readmissions) in the more affluent, better structured middle-class areas and the higher unduplicated admission rates (mainly readmissions) from the less affluent, more fluidly structured lower-class areas.

The most direct evidence to test this hypothesis must be case evidence taken on a person longitudinally over a long period of time. This evidence we do not have, but some studies using this and alternative procedures are referred to in Chapter 1. The evidence for a drift or social selection hypothesis, while not compelling, is still substantial.

This general line of reasoning is particularly applicable to schizophrenia, where we have noted that first admissions appear to be fairly randomly distributed throughout the city, crossing freely racial, ethnic, and socio-economic boundaries. The drift or social selection hypothesis has most usually been applied to the schizophrenic population, although it may well hold for the senile dementia patients as well. Schizophrenia is generally held to be the most chronic, disabling, and refractory of all mental disorders. Downward drift in the social structure after the onset of this disorder seems very likely in a competitive society which emphasizes superficial sociability, high earning power, and "making it." Our data also supports a drift phenomenon for senile dementia, but not for manic-depressive psychosis, psychoneurotic, psychophysiological, personality disorders or alcoholism.

Label Versus Disease

Consonant with previous studies, psychophysiological, psychoneurotic, and personality disorders appear to be diagnoses associated with the middle class. A similar situation obtains with the diagnosis of manic-depressive illness. The psychiatric epidemiologist is always faced with the problem of determining whether these disorders are really middle-class disorders or whether these labels get assigned to middle-class patients because they are somewhat more hopeful and agreeable than alternative diagnoses such as schizophrenia, senile dementia, and alcoholism. It is obvious that the data to definitively decide this issue is not present in this study. We can simply note that our data does, in fact, break diagnoses along socio-economic lines and express our own preference for a labelling hypothesis.

SUMMARY

This chapter has examined characteristics of Chicago communities and the relationship of these characteristics to utilization of mental hospitals by city residents. Each major diagnostic grouping was looked at in order to see if mental patients thus subdivided came from specific types of areas. For each diagnostic group, certain patterns emerged. Schizophrenia and senile and arterio-sclerotic psychoses are found to be associated with characteristic measures of socially unstable communities and with low economic status. The statistics on alcoholic admissions were harder to evaluate although there is a tendency for mental hospital alcoholics to come from the low-income areas with high percentages of substandard housing. With regard to schizophrenia, senile dementia, and alcoholism, the data appears to support a drift or social selection interpretation. The support for this contention lies in the finding that first admissions tend to come from more affluent, more socially structured communities, while unduplicated admissions (readmissions in particular) tend to emanate from poorer, less-structured communities.

NOTE

Dunham (1961) makes a case for social selection as a concept superior to and different from drift. However, the end product in any case would appear to be the same, i.e., the person moves downward socially and this downward movement is reflected in his choice of neighborhood in which to reside.

5. SPATIAL DISTRIBUTION OF MENTAL DISORDER IN CHICAGO

In looking at an urban area, the ecologist is interested in discovering whether spatial patterns occur among the several subcommunities in any specific urban area on the basis of some demographic and/or social problem indicators. In this chapter, we are concerned with plotting the spatial patterns of different diagnostic groups by patient's area of residence. This will be done, first, for all people admitted to public or private institutions during the study period; the data will then be divided into first admissions and readmissions to see if different spatial patterns occur for these subgroups.

UNDUPLICATED ADMISSIONS

Before looking at the various diagnostic patterns, a number of cautionary notes previously made should be re-emphasized. First, the patients in the sample do not include private or public facility outpatients, V. A. hospital patients, outpatients treated by private psychiatrists, or patients who received treatment outside of the State of Illinois. Second, the number of persons admitted for the first time to a mental hospital always underestimates true incidence. Similarly, total unduplicated admissions is an underestimate of prevalence. The number of persons readmitted during the study period refers to people who have had at least one admission to a public or private (inpatient) psychiatric institution prior to the study period. Third, psychiatric diagnoses tend to some extent to follow fashions and fads, have poor reliability, and are possibly related to class distance between therapist and patient (Hollingshead and Redlich, 1958). With these caveats in mind, let us proceed to see if geographical variation occurs among community areas with regard to admission rates.[1]

Map 3 shows the ecological distribution of unduplicated admissions to both public and private mental hospitals. The areas of high institutional utilization tend to be the areas around the central business district—the Loop (C.A. 32) and surrounding community areas. The Loop includes the skid-row section of Chicago as well as a number of major hotels and motels. The only major change in this downtown area of Chicago in recent years has been the building of a number of skyscraper office buildings after older buildings had been demolished. The building of skyscraper apartment and office buildings has continued apace in the Loop in the years since 1960.

Areas of high utilization are also noted in many lakeshore community areas from Rogers Park (C.A. 1) on the north side to South Shore (C.A. 43) on the south side. The lakefront community areas are generally characterized by heterogeneous populations both socially and economically, as well as by a high degree of mobility.

Map 4 views schizophrenic unduplicated admissions by area of residence. The highest concentration of admissions is generally in the community areas surrounding the center of the city. With a few exceptions, schizophrenic admission patterns are higher in lower income areas. These few exceptions include Uptown (C.A. 3), which has a large poor Appalachian white population in addition to a more affluent white population along the lakeshore, Hyde Park (C.A. 41), which has the University of Chica-

Map 3—Unduplicated adult admission rates

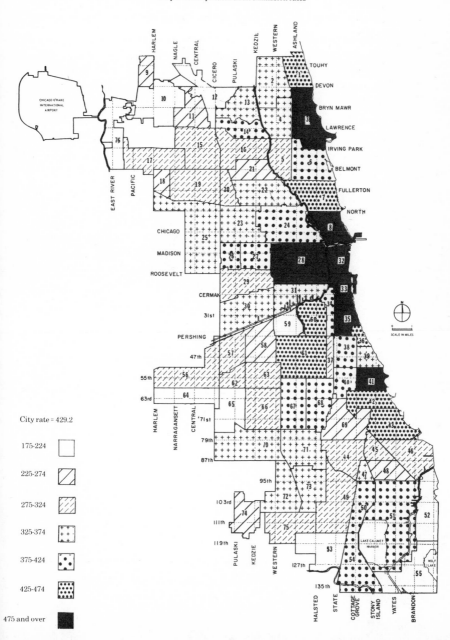

City rate = 429.2

175-224	
225-274	
275-324	
325-374	
375-424	
425-474	
475 and over	

Map 7—Unduplicated alcoholic adult admission rates

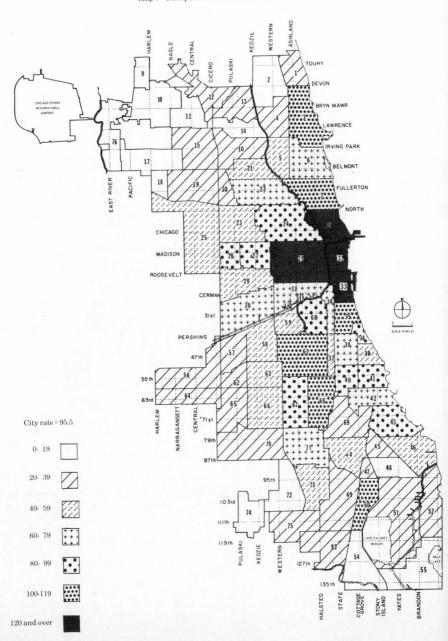

City rate = 95.5

0- 19

20- 39

40- 59

60- 79

80- 99

100-119

120 and over

go's faculty and student body, Burnside (C.A. 47) and New City (C.A. 61), which are lower middle class areas with a fairly high foreign stock composition.

Map 5 shows the distribution of people admitted to mental hospitals with a manic-depressive diagnosis. The high utilization areas are generally scattered over the city. One interesting pattern occurs in the northeastern community areas where there are three high-rate areas—Rogers Park (C.A. 1), West Ridge (C.A. 2), and Uptown (C.A. 3). In 1960, all three of these community areas had large Jewish populations. However, Uptown is more heterogeneous ethnically than either Rogers Park or West Ridge. There are a few southeastern community areas which also show fairly high rates. South Shore (C.A. 43) had a large middle class Jewish population in 1960; Avalon Park (C.A. 45) had a large middle class population with many first- and second-generation Americans; Roseland (C.A. 49) was racially, ethnically, and economically mixed in 1960; South Deering (C.A. 51) and Hegewisch (C.A. 55) were lower middle class blue-collar communities in 1960. Moreover, high-rate manic-depressive communities are much more difficult to interpret because of the small number of people being given this diagnosis.

Map 6 shows the distribution of cases with a diagnosis of senile psychosis or cerebral arteriosclerosis. An interesting pattern emerges in that almost all lakeshore community areas from the Near North Side (C.A. 8) to Woodlawn (C.A. 42), and a number of community areas immediately west of these areas, show high utilization rates. An exception to this pattern is Hyde Park (C.A. 41). Other high utilization areas are scattered over the city. Intuitively it would be expected that this diagnostic grouping would come from areas where there is a large proportion of people over 65 years of age, i.e., as the percentage of elderly people in a community area increases,

Map 5—Unduplicated manic-depressive psychoses adult admission rates

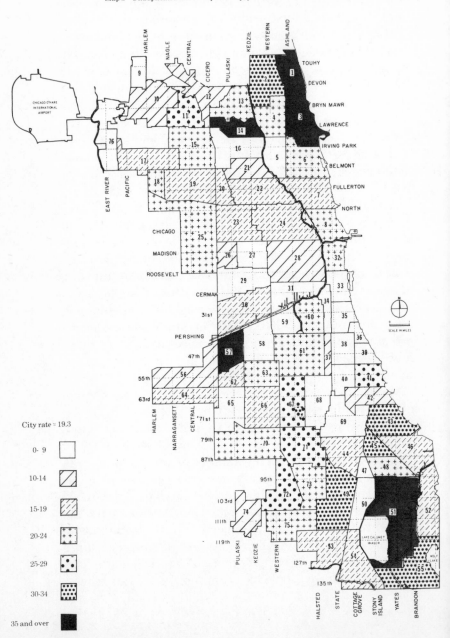

City rate = 19.3

0- 9

10-14

15-19

20-24

25-29

30-34

35 and over

Map 6—Unduplicated senile and arteriosclerotic admission rates

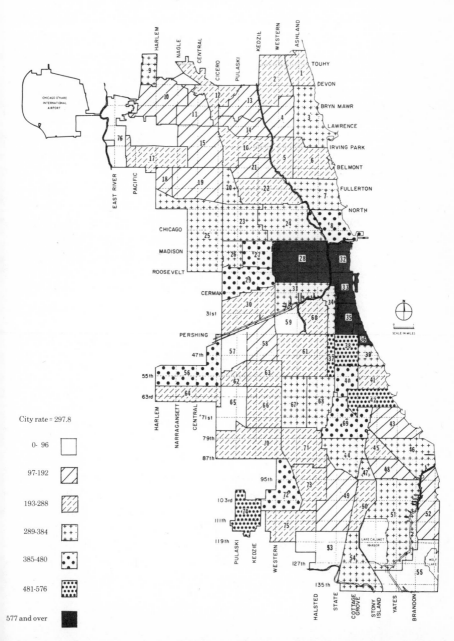

City rate = 297.8

0- 96

97-192

193-288

289-384

385-480

481-576

577 and over

the utilization rate for those patients with a diagnosis of senile dementia or cerebral arteriosclerosis should also increase. In computing an ecological correlation, an inverse relationship was found between these two variables (r = -0.45). Thus, the percentage of elderly people in the community does not appear to be related to utilization of inpatient psychiatric facilities. However, there is a 0.72 correlation between senile and arteriosclerotic admissions and percent of people in the community area with income under $3,000 a year, firmly establishing the link between poverty and mental hospital admission for a disease of the senium.

Alcoholic admissions are recorded in Map 7. The highest utilization rates occur around the central business district. Other high areas include Uptown (C.A. 3) with a heterogeneous social and economic population, Pullman (C.A. 50) with a large Italian population, New City (C.A. 61) with heterogeneous ethnic groups, and Englewood (C.A. 68) with a large black population.

Map 8 shows the distribution of psychophysiologic, psychoneurotic, and other personality disorders. The major difficulty in looking at ecological patterning for these disorders is that people with nonpsychotic diagnoses tend to use outpatient rather than inpatient services. Despite this limitation, however, a substantial number of persons were admitted to mental hospitals from Chicago with diagnoses of PP, PN, and PD. There is one interesting pattern in the north lakeshore community areas and extreme northeast community areas where high rates of mental hospital utilization occur. These areas tend to be quite heterogeneous on the whole but tend to have large middle class populations. The major exceptions to this generalization are the community areas close to the Loop (C.A. 32), i.e., Near North Side (C.A. 8), which is heterogeneous in racial and cultural composition but poorer than the northeastern communi-

Map 4—Unduplicated schizophrenic adult admission rates

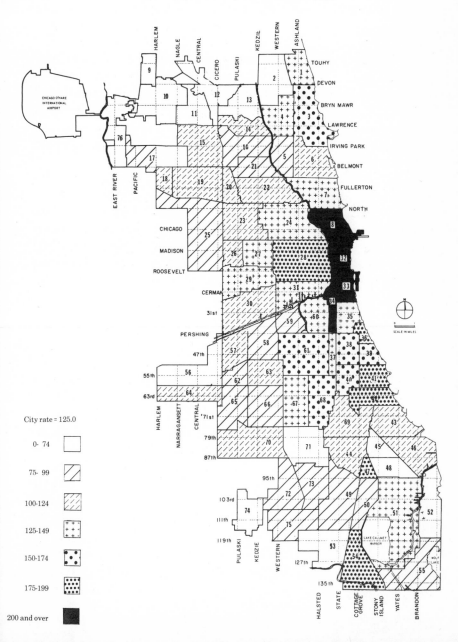

Map 8—Unduplicated psychophysiologic, psychoneurotic, and personality disorder adult admission rates

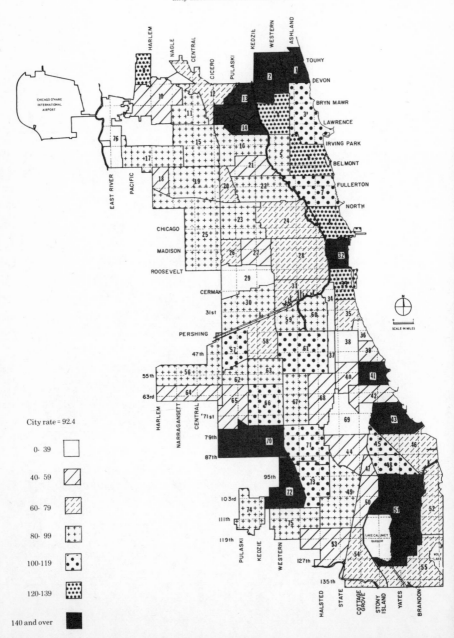

City rate = 92.4

0- 39

40- 59

60- 79

80- 99

100-119

120-139

140 and over

ty areas, and the Near South Side (C.A. 33), which is a poor black area but includes a large private hospital within its confines. Other high-rate areas are scattered but tend to be primarily middle class.

FIRST ADMISSIONS
AND READMISSIONS

Faris and Dunham's study on mental disorders in Chicago was based on data related to all new cases (first admissions) admitted to four State of Illinois mental institutions, and a small number of private mental institutions, from 1922 through 1934. The present study includes information on all public and private Illinois mental institutions which accepted city of Chicago people during a one-year period. Thus the present study is not a replication of the original study. However, it is still possible to make comparisons between the two studies on the basis of the spatial patterns of first admissions.

In this section, first admissions and readmissions will be viewed spatially with regard to diagnosis. First admissions plus readmissions add up to the unduplicated admissions presented in the first part of this chapter. Map 9 shows the spatial distribution of all first admissions regardless of diagnosis. The highest utilization areas still tend to be the areas in the center of the city. However, the pattern is not as strong as for unduplicated admissions. A number of high first admission rate areas can be found in the northeastern community areas and on the northwest and southwest perimeters of the city which are primarily middle class or with a strong middle class population component. Other high first admission rate areas are scattered over the city. Thus, it would appear that first admissions to cluster significantly in the city center but also can come from any area in the city and the areas

Map 9—Adult first admission rates

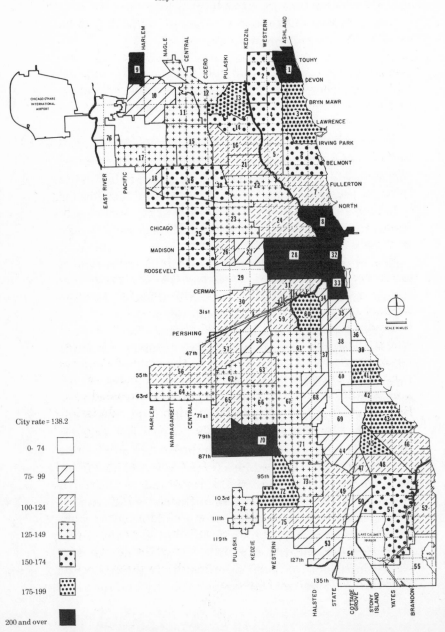

away from the city center tend to be of a higher socio-economic level generally than the central city areas.

Map 10 looks at readmissions without regard to diagnosis. The readmissions pattern is quite clear-cut. The highest rates are in the central city and its surrounding community areas to the west and north, and south along the lake-shore. These are the areas of physical deterioration and urban renewal. They are poorer areas which have a large number of social problems associated with them.

Whereas Faris and Dunham found first admission patterns generally to be highest in areas of high social disorganization, the present study finds first admission patterns as high in predominantly middle class areas. The data does suggest that as a mental illness progresses and repeated hospitalizations become necessary, people tend to relocate in the poorer areas of the city.

Map 11 looks at the pattern for first admission schizophrenics. No clear-cut pattern emerges. High first admission rate areas are scattered over the city. The characteristics of the high first admission rate areas vary. For example, Hyde Park (C.A. 41) is a community area in which there has been much urban renewal. As mentioned previously, Hyde Park is also the home of the University of Chicago. The median family income of the area was $6772 in 1959. This area can be contrasted with Beverly (C.A. 72) which is also a high first admission rate area. The area is upper middle class. The median family income in the area in 1959 was $11,437. Thus, community areas with a high rate of first admissions with a schizophrenic diagnosis are not necessarily low-income areas. This contrasts strongly with the finding in the Faris and Dunham study that the highest rates of first admission schizophrenia are to be found in the disorganized poor communities at or near the center of the city and diminish as one proceeds towards the north, west, and south peripheries of the city.

Map 10—Adult readmission rates

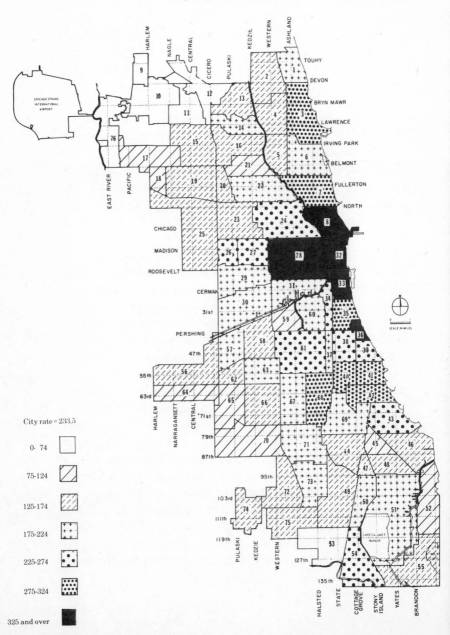

Map 11—Schizophrenic adult first admission rates

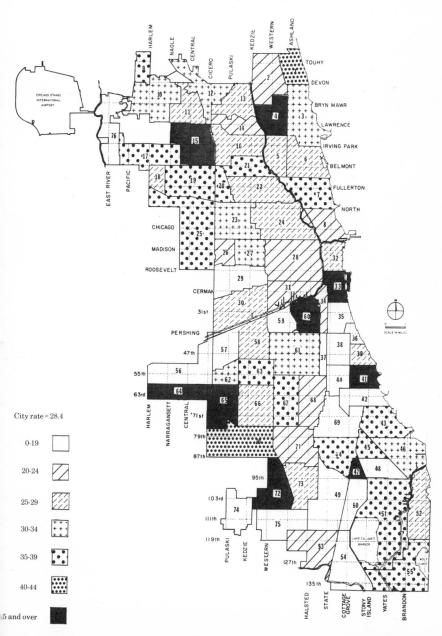

City rate = 28.4

0-19

20-24

25-29

30-34

35-39

40-44

5 and over

Map 12—Schizophrenic adult readmission rates

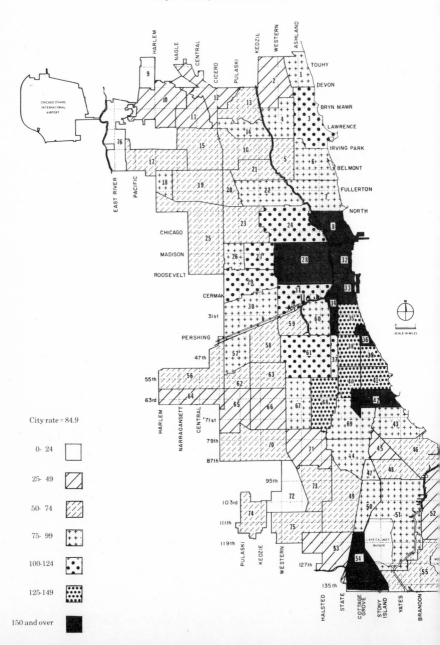

City rate = 84.9

0- 24	
25- 49	
50- 74	
75- 99	
100-124	
125-149	
150 and over	

Schizophrenic readmission patterns can be seen in Map 12. The readmission pattern is more clear-cut. Like the pattern for total readmissions, schizophrenic readmissions tend to come from the poorer community areas near the center of the city. We would hypothesize that drift has occurred because of the great difference between the first admission schizophrenic pattern and the readmission pattern.

Maps 13 and 14 look at the first admission and readmission manic-depressive patterns. The small number of cases with this diagnosis make interpretation difficult. First admissions, while quite scattered, seem to come primarily from middle class community areas.[2] Although not very strong, the readmission pattern seems stronger for the areas along the lakeshore. The meaning of this is not clear. The disorder has been associated with Jews and persons of eastern European stock; it has been negatively associated with being of Black racial stock. Our findings are generally in accord with these suggested characteristics of the disease.

The first admission pattern for senile and cerebral arteriosclerotic disease is very interesting (Map 15). High utilization areas are scattered and include middle class as well as poorer class community areas. It can be hypothesized that the first admission may be the only admission for many geriatric patients. If it were possible to superimpose a nursing home for the aged pattern over the mental hospital map, high rates of utilization might be found uniformly throughout the city. Map 16 shows high readmission rates for diseases of the senium in areas near the center of the city. This might be further evidence for support of a drift hypothesis with regard to this disorder.

The next two maps (17 and 18) show alcoholic patterns. The first admission pattern is quite strong. The highest areas of first admission tend to be at or near the

Map 13—Manic-depressive adult first admission rates

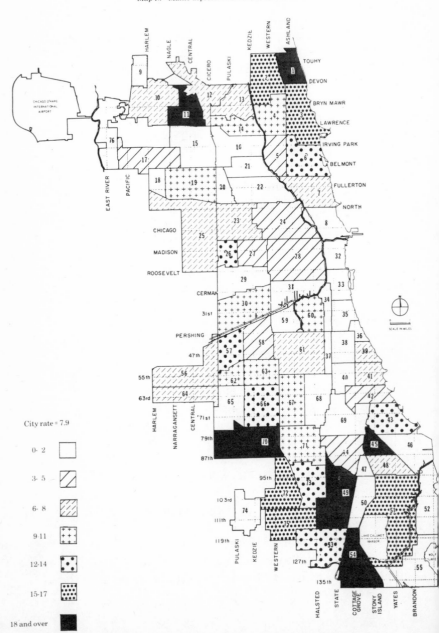

Map 14—Manic-depressive adult readmission rates

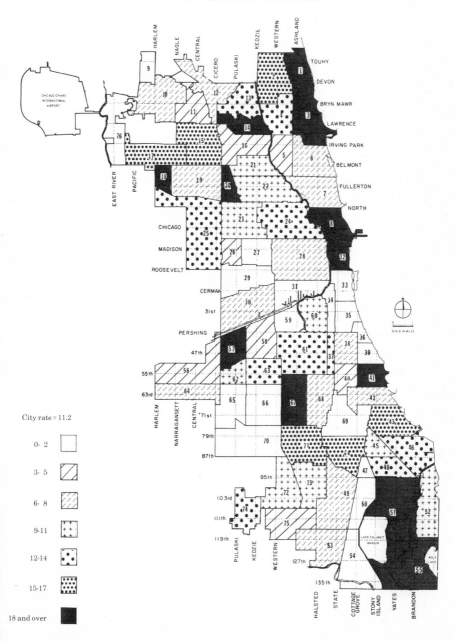

City rate = 11.2

0- 2

3- 5

6- 8

9-11

12-14

15-17

18 and over

Map 15—Senile and arteriosclerotic first admission rates

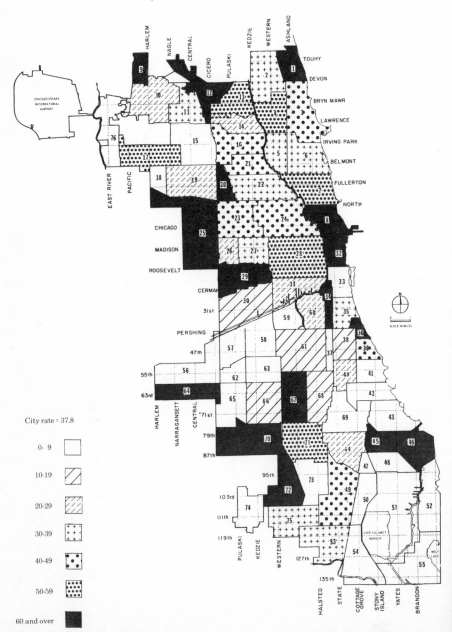

City rate = 37.8

0- 9

10-19

20-29

30-39

40-49

50-59

60 and over

Map 16—Senile and arteriosclerotic readmission rates

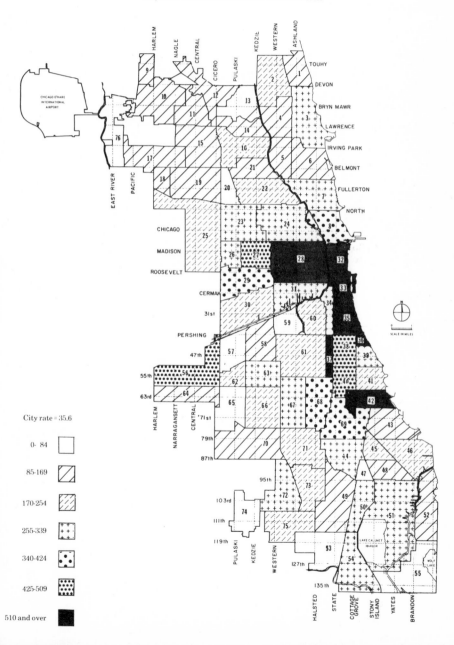

City rate = 35.6

0- 84	
85-169	
170-254	
255-339	
340-424	
425-509	
510 and over	

Map 17—Alcoholic adult first admission rates

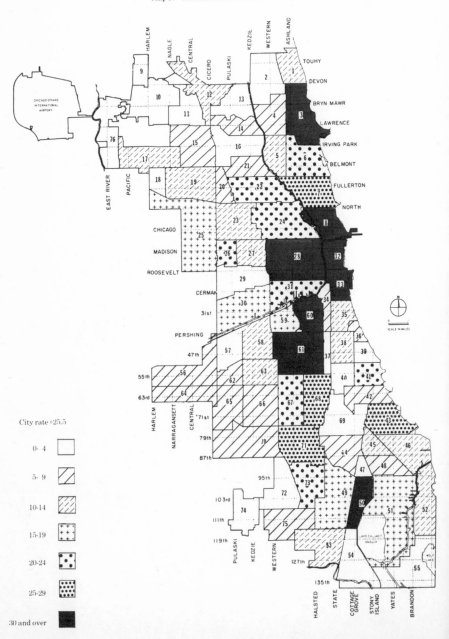

City rate =25.5

0- 4

5- 9

10-14

15-19

20-24

25-29

30 and over

Map 18—Alcoholic adult readmission rates

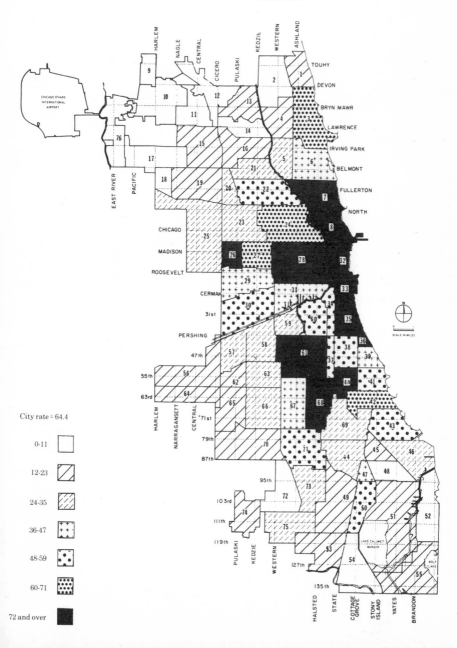

City rate = 64.4

0-11	
12-23	
24-35	
36-47	
48-59	
60-71	
72 and over	

Map 19—Psychophysiologic, psychoneurotic, and
personality disorder adult first admission rates

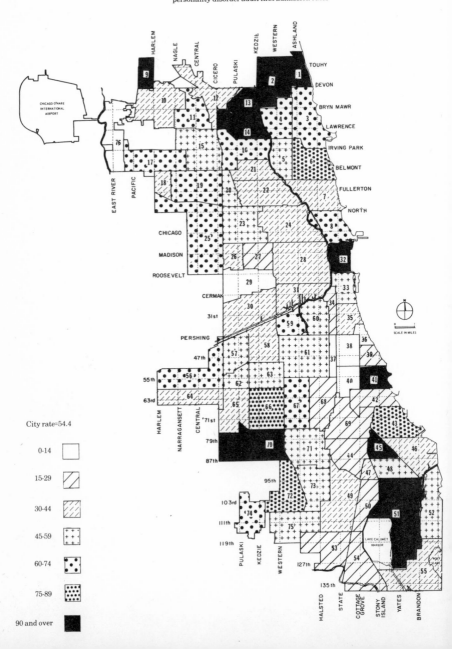

City rate=54.4

0-14

15-29

30-44

45-59

60-74

75-89

90 and over

Map 20—Psychophysiologic, psychoneurotic, and
personality disorder adult readmission rates

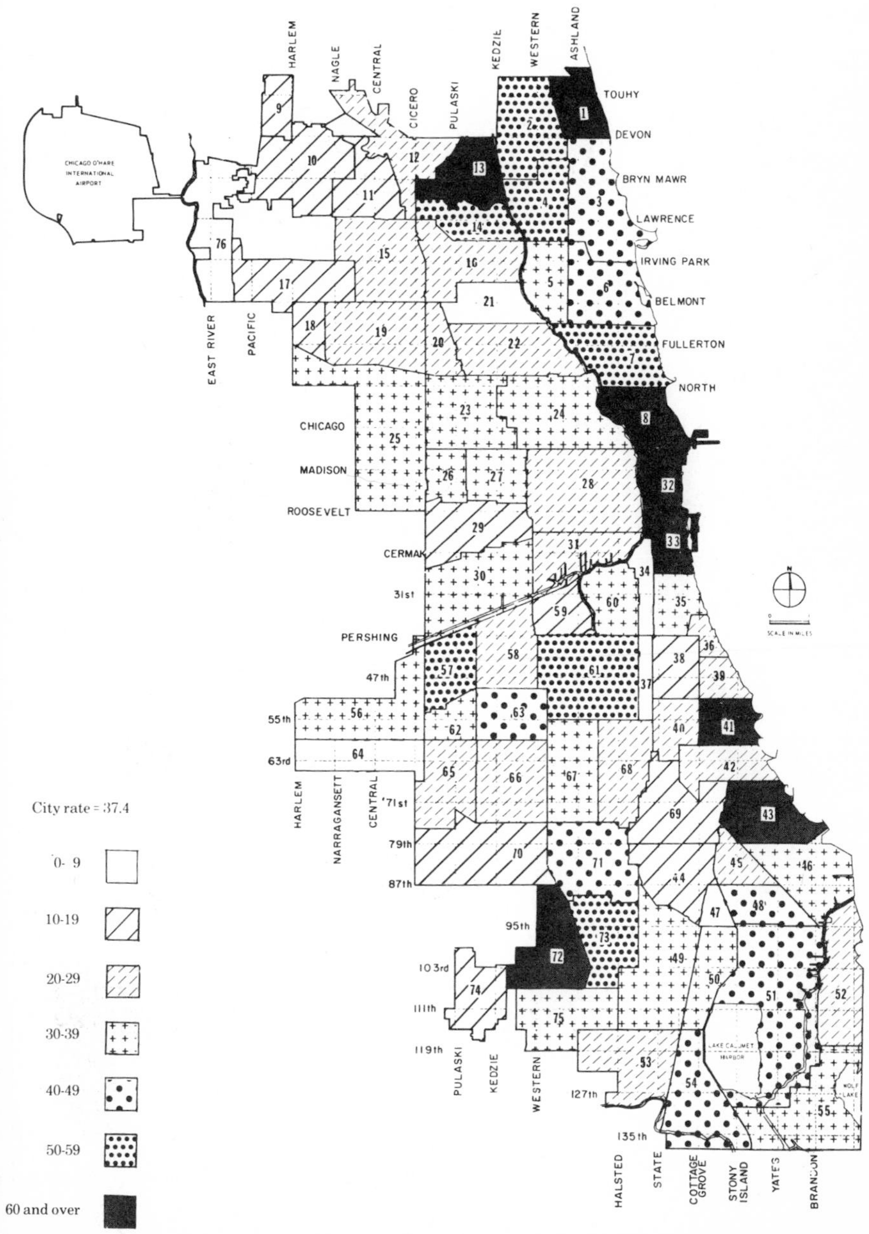

City rate = 37.4

0- 9

10-19

20-29

30-39

40-49

50-59

60 and over

center of the city, although there are exceptions. Uptown (C.A. 3) has a high first admission rate. As previously mentioned, Uptown had an extremely heterogeneous population in 1960 which included not only large white southern mountain and American Indian segments, but also Eskimos, European Jews, and other ethnic groups. The other noncentral city area which shows a high first admission rate is Pullman (C.A. 50) which is a lower middle class area with a fairly large foreign stock (Italians and Poles). The readmission pattern is similar to the first admission pattern for alcoholism with the central city community areas showing the highest rates.

The final two maps (19 and 20) show the spatial pattern for the nonpsychotic diagnoses. The high first admission areas are scattered over the city although there is a fairly strong pattern in the northeastern community areas. The high-rate areas generally are middle class or have a strong middle class component. The readmission pattern is interesting in that the lakeshore community areas north of the Loop (C.A. 32) show fairly high utilization. Most of these areas have a social and economic heterogeneity. Other high-rate areas are scattered throughout the city.

CONCLUSIONS

In this chapter, spatial patterning has been examined for the various psychiatric diagnostic groupings. Patterning in first admissions is not as clear-cut as it was when Faris and Dunham did their study. Communities are no longer as homogeneous or stable as they were in the twenties and thirties. Intercity expressways and industrial development have changed the geography of many community areas. Other changes from 1930 to 1960 concern the proliferation of general hospital beds for psychiatric patients and the increasing availability of health insurance covering mental illness.

A number of maps have been presented showing spatial patterning by place of residence for admissions to public and private mental institutions by city of Chicago people from July 1, 1960 to June 30, 1961. When the entire study population with a schizophrenic diagnosis was viewed, a pattern emerged similar to the first admission pattern found by Faris and Dunham. Schizophrenic unduplicated admissions were generally higher in low-income areas. The highest rates were found in the community areas surrounding the Loop in the city center and the community areas along the lakeshore.

In looking at the study population classified as first admission schizophrenic, no clear-cut pattern emerged. Thus, the pattern which Faris and Dunham found for first admission schizophrenics is not found in Chicago in 1961, although it is possible that trend data might display better patterns than were found in our data. Since the number and accessibility of general hospital psychiatric units has vastly increased from the 1930's to the present, the possibility exists that in the twenties and thirties poor (first admission) schizophrenics went to state hospitals but middle class schizophrenics either went to private sanitaria (often outside the state) or simply were kept at home. Today, because of the easier availability of general hospital psychiatric units and somewhat lessened shame and stigma, the "latent" middle class schizophrenic population is being recorded. Thus a more even distribution of admissions over the city is seen because middle class areas are more properly represented in our study. One should go further to note that since the unduplicated admissions of schizophrenia do approximate the Faris and Dunham pattern, this may conform to a drift or social selection hypothesis; as schizophrenics proceed through their subsequent admissions they may be aggregating in the poor city center which is the same locus of poverty and social disorganization as it was in the twenties and thirties.

As regards the manic-depressive diagnosis, no strong pattern was found. Generally, first admissions appear to come from middle class areas. This finding is similar to the Faris and Dunham conclusions on this disorder.

Faris And Dunham found that alcoholic psychoses and senile psychoses demonstrate patterns similar to schizophrenia with the highest rates in or near the center of the city. Our data support Faris and Dunham on the alcoholic psychoses but not on the first admission senile psychoses where cases seem to come from poor as well as socially more affluent areas. However, the readmission pattern seems to approximate the Faris and Dunham pattern.

Similar to the findings of Hollingshead and Redlich (1958), the nonpsychotic diagnoses tend to be reserved for people from middle class areas. The readmission pattern is interesting in that utilization rates are highest in areas undergoing much social change and areas which are socially heterogeneous in composition; this possibly reflects higher levels of social stress which may elevate the rate of psychoneurotic disorder.

NOTES

1. The tabular data is presented in Tables B-6 through B-10 in Appendix B.

2. Riverdale (C.A. 54) appears on the map as a high rate first admission area. This is very misleading. There is only one case with a manic-depressive diagnosis. However, since the adult population base of the community is so small (4941), the rate is greatly inflated.

6. ADMISSIONS BY TYPE OF INSTITUTION

Up to now, little consideration has been given to the differences in utilization rates by type of institution. For the present study, as was pointed out earlier, information on hospital utilization was gathered from all thirteen State of Illinois mental hospitals, eighteen general hospitals with psychiatric units, and thirteen private psychiatric hospitals and sanitaria. From all available information, these institutions were the only institutions in Illinois which accepted city of Chicago admissions during the study period. Our study does not include people who utilized federal hospitals, e.g. Veterans Administration Hospitals, or hospitals in other states. Thus, our study population is underrepresented as regards these latter institutions.

This chapter will be concerned with a consideration of the public and private institutions by area of residence of patients. The data are reported, first, on the basis of all people admitted, and, second, on the basis of first admissions only.

UNDUPLICATED ADMISSIONS

Of the 10,653 people admitted to the forty-four institutions studied, 6,725 people were admitted to state hospitals (63%); 2,404 were admitted to psychiatric units of general hospitals (23%); and 1,524 were admitted to private psychiatric hospitals and sanitaria (14%). The admission rate per 100,000 adult population 15 years of age and

91

over was 429.2. The utilization rates per 100,000 adult population for public and private institutions were as follows:

(1) 270.9 for state hospitals;
(2) 61.4 for private institutions;
(3) 96.9 for psychiatric units of general hospitals.

Using these city-wide rates it is then possible to see if any given community area falls above or below the city-wide rate (Table B-11 in Appendix B). In order to see the geographic variation between community areas with regard to admissions rates, a number of statistical maps are again employed. Map 21 looks at unduplicated admissions to state hospitals per 100,000 adult population. The areas of high institutional utilization tend to be the areas around the central business district (C.A. 32). These areas tend to be sociologically heterogeneous. There are some interesting exceptions to the general pattern for high utilization areas. Hermosa (C.A. 20) is primarily a middle class community area but there were signs in 1960 of the beginnings of housing deterioration and social change. Between 1930 and 1960, the population of the area had been slowly but progressively declining. Very little construction occurred after 1950. However, almost half of the community was composed of first- and second-generation American families in 1960. Riverdale (C.A. 54) also shows high utilization. This area was primarily black (90%) in 1960 with a large percentage of low-income families (46.8%). This area is largely composed of public housing.

Map 22 looks at unduplicated admissions to private mental institutions. The strongest pattern can be seen in the northside community areas, which tend to be middle class communities or to have a large middle class component. There are also some high-rate areas in the southeast section of Chicago. These areas tend to be lower middle class communities.

Map 21—Unduplicated adult admission rates
to Illinois state mental hospitals

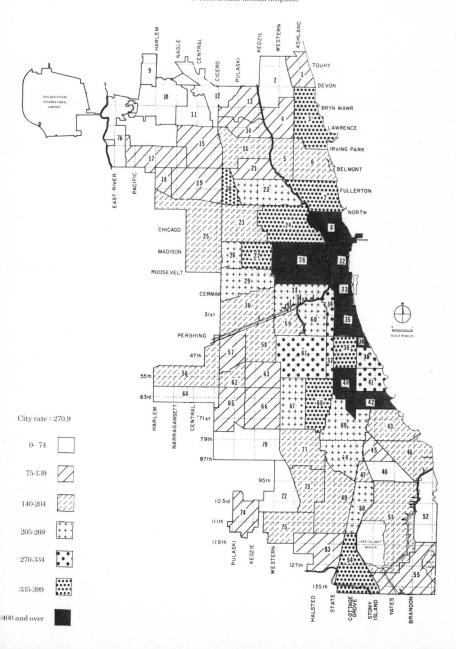

City rate = 270.9

0- 74

75-139

140-204

205-269

270-334

335-399

400 and over

Map 22—Unduplicated adult admission rates
to private mental hospitals

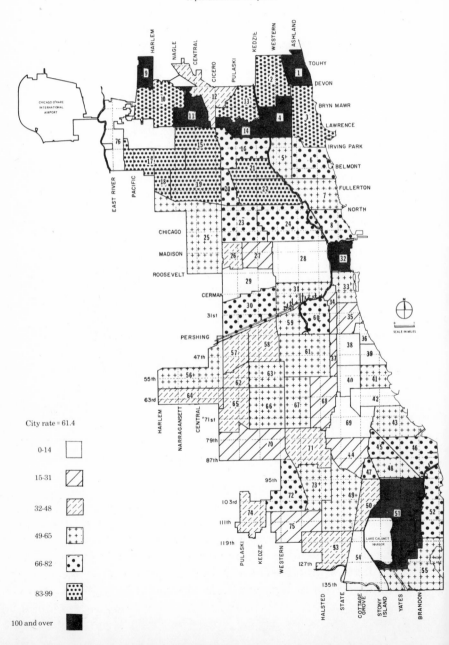

City rate = 61.4

0-14

15-31

32-48

49-65

66-82

83-99

100 and over

The use of psychiatric units of general hospitals is more spread out over the city than admissions to private mental institutions (Map 23). However, the high-utilization areas tend to be like the high-rate private institution areas sociologically in that they are primarily middle class areas.

FIRST ADMISSIONS

Of the 10,653 Chicago people admitted between July 1, 1960 and June 30, 1961, 3,431 or 32.2% were first admissions. The utilization rate for Chicago first admissions is 138.2 per 100,000 adult population (See Table B-12).

The over-all city rates per 100,000 adult population for public and private institutions were as follows:

(1) 38.3 for state hospitals;

(2) 38.7 for private institutions;

(3) 61.2 for psychiatric units of general hospitals.

The pattern for first admissions to state mental hospitals can be seen in Map 24. High state hospital first admission areas are found in community areas around the central business district where rates much higher than the city rate prevail. Areas which are low in first admissions to state hospitals cover the gamut from a low socioeconomic black area with a high delinquency rate, such as North Lawndale (C.A. 29), to middle class areas such as Rogers Park (C.A. 1) and Norwood Park (C.A. 10). Each community area would have to be looked at separately to explain the sociological and psychological reasons for a given amount of public mental hospital utilization at the time of first admission.

The highest rates of first admission to private mental institutions (Map 25) tend to be northside community areas with several exceptions. Regardless of location, high-rate areas tend to be middle class or to have a large percentage of middle-class residents. An interesting anomaly occurs in Uptown (C.A. 3) which has high ad-

Map 23—Unduplicated adult admission rates
to psychiatric units of general hospitals

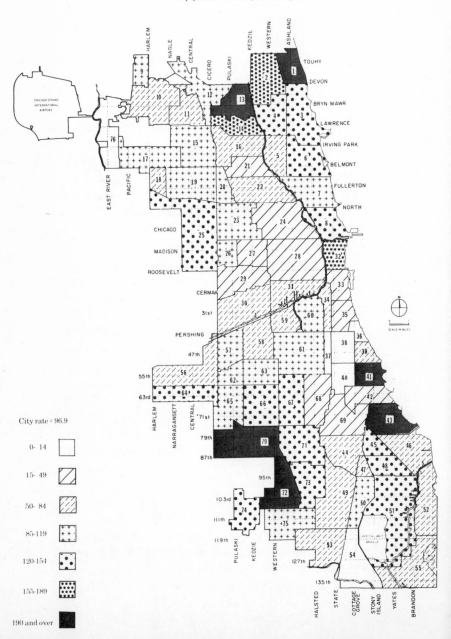

City rate = 96.9

0- 14

15- 49

50- 84

85-119

120-154

155-189

190 and over

Map 24—Adult first admission rates
to Illinois State mental hospitals

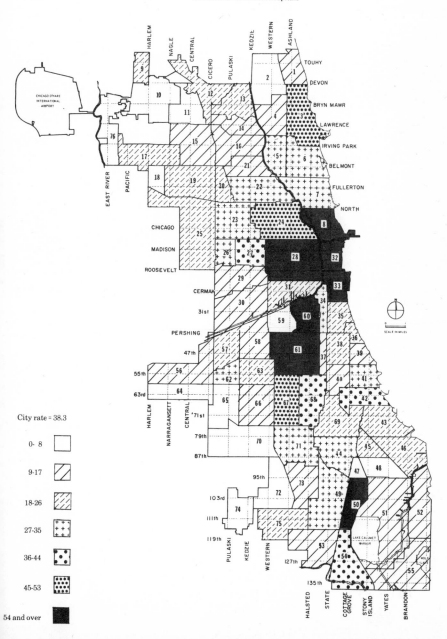

City rate = 38.3

0- 8	
9-17	
18-26	
27-35	
36-44	
45-53	
54 and over	

Map 25—Adult first admission rates
to private mental hospitals

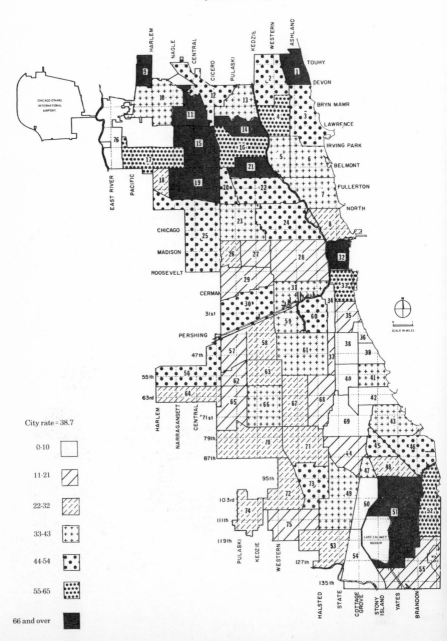

City rate = 38.7

0-10

11-21

22-32

33-43

44-54

55-65

66 and over

Map 26—Adult first admission rates
to psychiatric wards of general hospitals

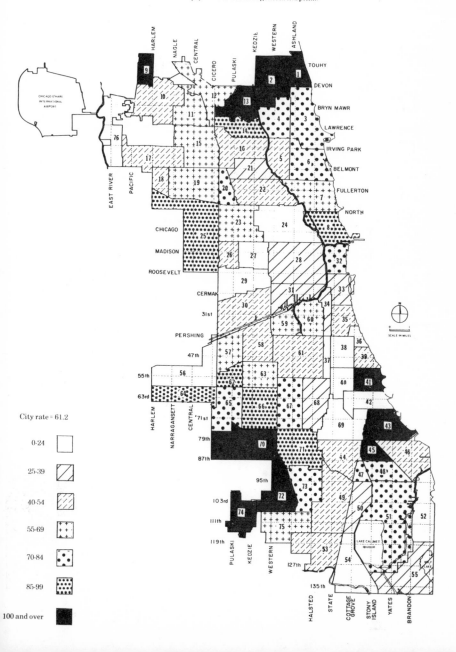

City rate = 61.2

0-24

25-39

40-54

55-69

70-84

85-99

100 and over

mission rates to both public and private institutions. This is probably due to the social heterogeneity of the area in which both high- and low-income groups and many ethnic minority groups can be found.

The largest percentage of first admissions utilize psychiatric units of general hospitals. Map 26 looks at the utilization pattern for these admissions. The pattern is not clear-cut. High utilization pockets can be seen in the northeastern community areas and the southwestern community areas. A few high-rate areas can also be seen in the southeastern sector of the city.

COMPARATIVE ANALYSIS

In order to see whether admissions to public and private institutions come from the same geographic areas, a correlation technique was employed (See Table 7). There is almost no relationship between the use of a state mental hospital and a psychiatric unit of a general hospital by place of residence for first admissions. Thus factors other than place of residence affect initial use of a mental hospital. For example, socio-economic considerations or family cohesiveness might well be more crucial.

The correlations between private institution utilization and psychiatric general hospital utilization tend to be strongly related for first admissions. This is not surprising in that the high-rate areas for both types of institution tend to be middle class and sociologically homogeneous. Other correlations not included in Table 7 show similar utilization patterns for unduplicated admissions.

SUMMARY

Sixty-three percent of the people admitted to inpatient facilities in Chicago in fiscal year 1961 went to state mental hospitals. However, only twenty-eight percent of the first admissions went to state mental hospitals. Forty-four percent of the first admissions went to psychiatric units of general hospitals.

With regard to all people admitted, the relationship between use of a public or private facility and the place of residence of admissions seems to be affected by factors other than residential location. This finding is also substantiated for first admissions. However, middle class homogeneous community areas will use private psychiatric hospitals as well as psychiatric units of general hospitals when service is needed. The state hospital pattern for these areas is not consistent.

The areas with high over all public and private hospital utilization tend to be areas surrounding the central business district and the community areas along the lakeshore. These are areas which today are undergoing a great deal of social change. Furthermore, they are areas which are characterized by heterogeneous populations.

7. ECOLOGICAL ATTRIBUTES OF HIGH AND LOW RATE MENTAL HOSPITAL UTILIZATION AREAS

This chapter is concerned with a detailed analysis of the ecological attributes of low-rate and high-rate admission areas in the city. High-rate areas are here defined as those with an unduplicated admission rate of 525+ per hundred thousand adult population during the study period; low-rate areas refer to community areas with an admission rate of 225 or less per hundred thousand adult population (See Map 27).

Using these cutting points, we find six high-rate areas. These are: the Loop (C.A. 32); three areas surrounding the Loop, the Near North Side, the Near West Side, and the Near South Side (C.A. 8, 28, and 33); and two lake-front communities, Uptown in the north (C.A. 3) and Hyde Park in the south (C.A. 41). It was decided to exclude the Loop (C.A. 32) from further analysis because it is a highly atypical area with a small resident population and an astonishing admission rate of 5584/100,000, a rate some thirteen times the city average. The Loop is the central business district of Chicago. Residentially, the area is quite transient. It includes the major hotels, theatres, and restaurants, as well as a skid-row area. The Loop and its three adjacent areas to the north, south, and

103

Map 27—High and low unduplicated admission rate areas

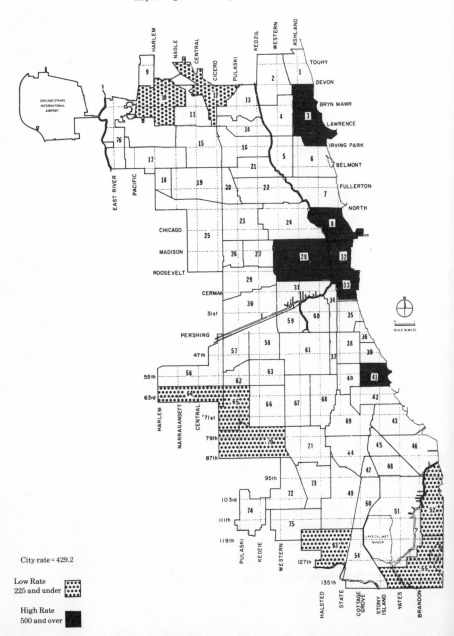

City rate = 429.2

Low Rate
225 and under

High Rate
500 and over

west constitute the city center and stand out clearly as the high psychiatric casualty rate areas of the city, with admission rates for all four areas in excess of 750/100,000. The two remaining high-rate areas, Hyde Park (C.A. 41) and Uptown (C.A. 3), while highly productive of psychiatric casualties, still rank a good distance below the city center areas with rates of 530/100,000 and 540/100,000 respectively.

The seven low-rate areas are located on the outlying perimeter of the city (semi-suburban areas). They are: Norwood Park (C.A. 10) and Forest Glen (C.A. 12) on the north; and Clearing (C.A. 64), West Lawn (C.A. 65), West Pullman (C.A. 53), Hegewisch (C.A. 55), and East Side (C.A. 52) on the south side of the city.

Table 9 arrays data on sex, race, age, and community growth characteristics for the five high- and seven low-rate areas. The sex distribution for the high- and low-rate areas is approximately equal. The low-rate areas contain very few blacks, under 0.5% in any of these areas. All high-rate areas, except Uptown, have a higher percentage of blacks than the reported 1960 city-wide average of 23%.

The age characteristics of the high- and low-rate areas show some interesting variations. Three high-rate areas show a large concentration of older persons (10-15%) and a concomitant smaller concentration of young people (20-26%) in comparison with the low-rate areas where representation of young persons ranges from 28-36% of the population and the aged account for 4-10%. The Near West Side and the Near South Side show some variance from the other high-rate areas with regard to age. Both of these areas are preponderantly black. Over 40% of the population of these two communities was under 18 in 1960. The concentration of older persons in these two areas approximates the low-rate areas. If a generalization can be made with regard to age, it would be that

TABLE 9
Sex, Race, Age, and Growth Characteristics of High and Low Rate Mental Hospital Utilization Areas in 1960

Community Areas	Total Population #	Total Population %	Sex[a] Male #	Sex[a] Male %	Sex[a] Female #	Sex[a] Female %	Race[b] White #	Race[b] White %	Race[b] Negro #	Race[b] Negro %	Age % 18 & Under	Age % 65 & Over	% Change 1950-1960[b] Total Population	% Change 1950-1960[b] Total Negro Population
High Rate Community Areas														
3 Uptown	127,682	100.0	60,673	47.5	67,009	52.5	122,595	96.0	423	0.3	20.5	14.8	- 8.2	-19.7
8 Near North Side	75,509	100.0	38,031	50.4	37,478	49.6	50,569	67.0	23,114	30.6	26.2	10.2	-15.3	29.8
28 Near West Side	126,610	100.0	67,056	53.0	59,554	47.0	57,676	45.6	68,146	53.8	40.5	5.8	-21.0	4.0
33 Near South Side	10,350	100.0	5,248	50.7	5,102	49.3	2,354	22.7	7,942	76.8	42.9	8.1	- 8.5	1.4
41 Hyde Park	45,577	100.0	21,970	48.2	23,607	51.8	27,214	59.7	17,163	37.7	23.4	11.6	-17.4	876.8
Low Rate Community Areas														
10 Norwood Park	40,953	100.0	19,857	48.5	21,096	51.5	40,915	99.9	12	0.0	31.7	9.0	52.8	—
12 Forest Glen	19,228	100.0	9,180	47.7	10,048	52.3	19,203	99.9	6	0.0	28.5	9.6	57.8	—
52 East Side	23,214	100.0	11,758	50.7	11,456	49.4	23,191	99.9	4	0.0	32.7	8.0	7.4	—
53 West Pullman	35,397	100.0	17,465	49.3	17,793	50.7	35,328	99.8	62	0.2	34.3	8.9	21.0	—
55 Hegewisch	8,936	100.0	4,602	51.5	4,334	48.5	8,900	99.6	32	0.4	34.7	7.5	25.1	—
64 Clearing	18,797	100.0	9,518	50.6	9,279	49.4	18,777	99.9	2	0.0	36.5	4.8	77.5	—
65 West Lawn	26,910	100.0	13,226	49.2	13,684	50.9	26,893	100.0	5	0.0	32.9	7.5	86.1	—

SOURCES:

[a]U.S. Bureau of the Census. U.S. Censuses of Population and Housing: 1960. Census Tracts. Final Report PHC (1) -26. Table P-2.

[b]E. M. Kitagawa and K. E. Taeuber. Local Community Fact Book: Chicago Metropolitan Area, Chicago: University of Chicago Press, Chicago Community Inventory, 1963.

there is a tendency for the high-rate areas to have older populations than the low-rate areas. This generalization is weakened by the difference noted on the Near West and Near South Sides. One should note that the Near West and Near South Sides are the site of large public housing projects which typically house families with a large number of younger children and adolescents.

Whereas all five of the high-rate areas show a decline in population between 1950 and 1960, all the low-rate areas show increases in population during the same period. These increases are substantial, ranging up to 86.1% in West Lawn (C.A. 65). All of the low-rate areas show increases in population in excess of 20% except East Side, which registers 7.4%. High-rate areas show a black in-migration between 1950 and 1960, except Uptown, where a substantial loss of 19.7% occurred. Hyde Park registered a phenomenal increase in black population of 877%.

Nativity characteristics are arrayed in Table 10. With two exceptions, low-rate areas have a higher percentage of foreign born than high-rate areas. However, the high-rate areas of Uptown and Hyde Park also have a high percentage of foreign born. When data for the first two generations (foreign born and native born with foreign or mixed parentage) are combined, the tendency for the low-rate areas to have a higher percentage of foreign stock than high-rate areas is strengthened. Low-rate areas are substantially composed of second-generation Americans. The high-rate area of Uptown tends to approximate the pattern noted in the low-rate areas. However, Uptown differs from the low-rate areas in that the ethnic composition of the area is more diversified than the low-rate areas. Uptown has a large American Indian population, a Japanese-American population, and a southern-mountain white population which accentuates the ethnic heterogeneity of the area.

TABLE 10

Nativity Percentages of High and Low Rate
Mental Hospital Utilization Areas in 1960

		Nativity Percentage		
High Rate Community Areas	Total Percent	Foreign Born	Native: Foreign or Mixed Parentage	Native: Native Parentage
3 Uptown	100.0	16.7	24.9	58.4
8 Near North Side	100.0	7.7	12.6	79.7
28 Near West Side	100.0	7.5	10.5	82.0
33 Near South Side	100.0	3.1	3.1	93.8
41 Hyde Park	100.0	11.0	16.0	73.0
Low Rate Community Areas				
10 Norwood Park	100.0	10.2	33.7	56.1
12 Forest Glen	100.0	10.8	34.9	54.3
52 East Side	100.0	11.5	31.1	57.4
53 West Pullman	100.0	12.7	33.2	54.1
55 Hegewisch	100.0	12.7	32.0	55.3
64 Clearing	100.0	8.1	28.3	63.6
65 West Lawn	100.0	10.9	35.5	53.6

Source: E. M. Kitagawa and K. E. Taeuber, *Local Community Fact Book.*
Chicago Metropolitan Area, Chicago: University of Chicago Press,
Chicago Community Inventory, 1963.

Table 11 deals with marital status. There is a higher concentration of unmarried people (single, separated, divorced, and widowed) in high-rate areas than in low-rate areas. Conversely, there is a much higher percentage of married people in the low-rate areas than in the high-rate areas. These findings are also obtained when the sex characteristic is controlled.

Education, employment, and family income characteristics are arrayed in Table 12. The findings in education are somewhat ambiguous. On the whole, the differences between high- and low-rate areas on median number of school years completed are minimal. Two high-rate areas (Near West Side and Near South Side) with large poor black populations[1] and two low-rate areas (Hegewisch and East Side) with stable white working-class popula-

TABLE 11
Marital Status Percentages by Sex
for High and Low Rate
Mental Hospital Utilization Areas in 1960.

	Total Percentages					Female Percentages					Male Percentages				
	% Sin-gle	% Mar-ried	% Sep-arated	% Wid-owed	% Di-vorced	% Sin-gle	% Mar-ried	% Sep-arated	% Di-vorced	% Wid-owed	% Sin-gle	% Mar-ried	% Sep-arated	% Di-vorced	% Wid-owed
High Rate Community Areas															
3 Uptown	26.2	56.2	2.3	11.8	5.8	23.1	52.9	2.3	6.2	17.8	29.7	59.9	2.3	5.3	5.1
8 Near North Side	39.4	45.0	4.6	9.4	6.2	34.9	44.8	5.1	6.4	13.9	43.9	45.0	4.1	6.0	5.1
28 Near West Side	31.7	55.6	8.9	8.4	4.3	23.7	60.6	10.4	3.8	11.9	38.4	51.4	7.7	4.7	5.5
33 Near South Side	28.2	54.3	12.4	12.3	5.1	22.3	57.5	14.9	15.2	5.0	33.7	51.4	10.1	9.7	5.2
41 Hyde Park	30.6	54.4	4.3	9.8	5.2	26.7	52.5	5.2	5.9	14.9	35.0	56.5	3.3	4.4	4.1
Low Rate Community Areas															
10 Norwood Park	21.5	77.1	0.5	5.2	1.0	20.4	66.5	0.5	1.8	11.3	22.6	73.2	0.2	0.9	3.3
12 Forest Glen	21.6	70.0	0.4	7.3	1.1	21.1	66.4	0.5	1.4	11.1	22.2	74.0	0.3	0.7	3.1
52 East Side	23.5	66.8	0.8	7.5	2.3	19.1	67.1	0.9	2.2	11.3	27.6	66.4	0.7	2.3	3.7
53 West Pullman	21.2	70.8	0.8	5.7	1.8	18.6	67.9	1.0	2.1	11.4	24.0	70.3	0.6	1.9	3.8
55 Hegewisch	23.3	67.2	0.8	7.6	1.9	18.5	68.6	0.7	1.9	11.0	27.9	65.8	0.8	1.9	4.4
64 Clearing	21.6	69.1	0.8	7.7	2.0	18.3	71.1	0.9	2.1	8.5	24.8	70.6	0.6	1.6	3.0
65 West Lawn	21.2	70.1	0.7	7.2	1.5	19.3	68.3	0.9	1.7	10.7	23.3	72.1	0.4	1.2	3.4

Source: E. M. Kitagawa and K. E. Taeuber, *Local Community Fact Book: Chicago Metropolitan Area*, Chicago: University of Chicago Press, Chicago Community Inventory, 1963.

TABLE 12
Education, Employment, and Family Income Characteristics of High and Low Rate Mental Hospital Utilization Areas in 1960

	Education		Employment				Family Income		
Community Areas	Med. School Year Completed (1959)	Percent with 4 or more yrs. college	Percent of all workers in mfg.	Percent of all males in white-collar occ.	Percent of L.F. Unemployed	Med. Family Income	Med. Family Income	Percent with Income Under $3,000	Percent with Income Over $10,000
High Rate Community Areas									
3 Uptown	11.6	9.4	26.4	49.9	3.9	6,780		13.1	22.7
8 Near North Side	12.0	17.9	17.0	55.3	5.8	5,552		24.2	27.4
28 Near West Side	8.3	3.5	29.3	21.5	11.6	3,984		36.8	5.3
33 Near South Side	8.6	2.9	25.2	20.5	14.5	3,280		46.0	5.0
41 Hyde Park	12.5	26.7	17.1	62.3	5.1	6,772		13.8	26.3
Low Rate Community Areas									
10 Norwood Park	11.0	6.4	40.3	46.2	2.0	8,659		4.6	36.7
12 Forest Glen	12.2	13.7	31.4	68.2	1.7	11,116		3.8	56.6
52 East Side	9.5	2.0	51.9	20.1	4.1	7,370		7.1	24.1
53 West Pullman	10.3	3.6	40.0	30.9	3.4	7,496		8.1	24.2
55 Hegewisch	8.9	1.1	55.0	18.9	5.0	7,004		8.0	20.3
64 Clearing	10.2	3.6	46.2	29.4	3.1	7,584		5.1	24.8
65 West Lawn	10.3	2.9	41.7	32.4	2.2	7,900		4.5	28.2

Source: E. M. Kitagawa and K. E. Taeuber, *Local Community Fact Book: Chicago Metropolitan Area*, Chicago: University of Chicago Press, Chicago Community Inventory, 1963.

tions show the lowest median educational level of the 12 areas. The remaining high- and low-rate areas show a median educational level of between two and four years of high school. Median number of school years completed leaves a number of questions unanswered concerning the education variable. Some further light is shed on this variable when the percent with four or more years of college is examined. All but one of the low-rate areas (Forest Glen) show low concentrations of college graduates. Three of the high-rate areas (Hyde Park, Near North, and Uptown) show high concentrations of college graduates. The general trend is for high-rate areas to show a higher percentage of college graduates than low-rate areas. Hyde Park shows the highest concentration of college graduates of the twelve areas. This is a consequence of the fact that the University of Chicago is located in this community and faculty, by and large, tend to reside in the Hyde Park area rather than commute.

With the exception of the two high-rate areas with large poor black populations, the percent of white-collar workers is generally higher in high-rate areas than in low-rate areas. Norwood Park and Forest Glen, which are low-rate areas, do show large percentages of white-collar workers. However, the concentration of workers in manufacturing industries (blue-collar occupations) is consistently higher in low-rate areas than in high-rate areas. In addition, people who live in low-rate areas tend to be occupationally more stable than people in high-rate areas. Unemployment rates are generally higher in high-rate areas than in low-rate areas.

The median family income is higher in low-rate areas than in high-rate areas. Moreover, the percent of population with incomes under $3,000 a year in 1959 is markedly higher in high-rate areas than in low-rate areas. With the exception of the Near West and Near South Sides, the percent of population with an income exceeding $10,000

TABLE 13
Housing Characteristics of High and Low Rate
Mental Hospital Utilization Areas in 1960

Housing Data

Community Areas	Percent Built 1950 or later	Percent Owner Occupied	Percent Sub-standard Housing	Percent with more than one person per room	Med. value, Owner units in one unit structures	Med. Number of Rooms	Med. Gross Rent, Renter Units
High Rate Community Areas							
3 Uptown	4.8	9.3	20.5	9.1	19,000	2.9	91
8 Near North Side	14.5	6.0	34.8	12.8	25,000+	2.3	82
28 Near West Side	10.0	9.6	44.4	28.9	12,400	3.6	66
33 Near South Side	22.3	1.6	52.8	30.1	—	2.3	64
41 Hyde Park	2.7	9.5	13.9	9.6	18,800	3.2	100
Low Rate Community Areas							
10 Norwood Park	40.5	83.3	0.7	4.9	21,900	5.2	114
12 Forest Glen	45.1	87.1	0.6	2.5	25,000+	5.7	121
52 East Side	14.8	64.6	4.6	8.4	15,100	5.1	81
53 West Pullman	24.3	66.6	4.4	8.2	16,300	5.1	83
55 Hegewisch	29.2	67.0	6.0	11.9	14,400	4.8	73
64 Clearing	49.4	74.6	2.0	11.6	17,400	4.9	95
65 West Lawn	51.5	82.6	1.7	7.6	18,900	4.9	98

Source: E. M. Kitagawa and K. E. Taeuber, *Local Community Fact Book: Chicago Metropolitan Area*, Chicago: University of Chicago Press, Chicago Community Inventory, 1963.

per year does not differ radically in high- and low-rate areas.

Table 13 reports differences in housing characteristics between high- and low-rate areas. The high-rate areas contain older buildings, generally renter rather than owner occupied, and a large percentage of substandard housing. The low-rate areas show considerable construction of new buildings between 1950 and 1960. They are generally owner occupied and in good condition. The median number of rooms per house or apartment is generally higher in low-rate areas. Rents are lower in high-rate areas in comparison with low-rate areas, but the difference is not striking. With the exception of the Near West and Near South Sides, which are high-rate areas, there is no substantial difference in percentage of housing units with more than one person per room between the high- and low-rate areas. The two black ghetto areas show the greatest density per housing unit.

Table 14 presents data on juvenile delinquency, illegitimacy, and public assistance.[2] Utilizing the number of males brought to Family Court of Cook County in delinquency petitions as a measure of juvenile delinquency, it is apparent that the high-rate areas have higher rates of reported delinquency than the low-rate areas. Reported illegitimate births are strikingly higher in high-rate areas than in low-rate areas. As regards public assistance data, a negligible number of persons in low-rate areas are on public assistance, whereas there are substantial numbers on public assistance in high-rate areas. Thus, on these three social problem indicators, high-rate areas are substantially more problematic than low-rate areas. The high-rate areas tend to fit the social disorganization pattern which Faris and Dunham found in Chicago in the early 1930's.

Table 15 presents data on psychiatric diagnosis for unduplicated admissions. Schizophrenia rates are substantially higher in high-rate areas than in low-rate areas.

TABLE 14
Selected Social Problem Indicators of High and Low Rate Mental Hospital Utilization Areas

Community Areas	No. of Males brought before Family Court of Cook County on delinquency petitions 1958-1961		Illegitimate Births (1962)		Public Assistance (1962)	
	Number	Rate/100 Boys (12-16 yrs.)	Number	Percent of Live Births	Number	Recipients/100 Pop. (1960)
High Rate Community Areas						
3 Uptown	75	2.9	204	7.8	4,300	3.4
8 Near North Side	108	6.2	611	29.7	12,680	16.4
28 Near West Side	288	6.1	1,021	25.8	31,240	24.7
33 Near South Side	34	8.5	95	36.4	3,410	32.9
41 Hyde Park	33	3.5	89	10.5	2,110	4.6
Low Rate Community Areas						
10 Norwood Park	18	1.0	5	1.1	70	0.2
12 Forest Glen	4	0.6	2	1.2	10	0.1
52 East Side	18	1.9	5	1.3	200	0.9
53 West Pullman	20	1.3	11	2.3	450	1.3
55 Hegewisch	6	1.5	0	0.0	70	0.8
64 Clearing	13	1.7	6	2.0	20	0.1
65 West Lawn	10	0.9	7	2.9	60	0.2

Source: *Chicago Community Area Profiles*, Chicago: Welfare Council of Metropolitan Chicago, 1964.

The same communities which have high schizophrenic rates have high rates for senile and arteriosclerotic disease, alcoholism, and also psychophysiologic, psychoneurotic, and personality disorders (PP, PN, and PD). Manic-depressive illness rates differ from this pattern. The rates for this illness are highest in Uptown and Hyde Park, which are high-rate areas, and in Hegewisch, which is a low-rate area. The remaining areas do not differ greatly in the rates of hospital use for this disorder. Thus, with the exception of manic-depressive illness, one may observe that high-rate areas and low-rate areas are quite differentiated on all psychiatric diagnoses recorded when one looks at unduplicated admissions.

When one turns to a consideration of Table 16, which records first admissions by diagnosis, several interesting findings emerge. As one might expect, the areas that are high in total unduplicated admissions remain high in total first admissions; all are well above the city-wide average and in all cases are higher than the low rate unduplicated admission areas. However, when one looks at the first admission rates for specific diagnostic groups, the pattern is not uniform. For schizophrenia, the first admission rates are entirely comparable between the high- and low-rate areas. First admission schizophrenics are spread quite randomly over the city. It would appear that, although all Chicago communities have roughly similar rates of production of first admissions for schizophrenia, some communities appear to manage persons with such a disorder in such a way that the likelihood of subsequent and multiple hospitalization is drastically reduced. The same communities which have high extrusion rates (unduplicated admissions) for schizophrenics have, as noted above, high extrusion rates for senile and arteriosclerotic persons, alcoholics, and PP, PN, and PD. For the first admission data, the numbers of admissions for manic-depressive psychosis and for senile and arterio-

TABLE 15
Admissions by Selected Diagnoses for High and Low Rate Mental Hospital Utilization Areas

Community Areas	Total Population #	Rate	Schizo-phrenic #	Rate	Manic-Depressive #	Rate	Senile & Arterio. #	Rate	Alcoholic #	Rate	PP, PN, & PD. #	Rate
High Rate Community Areas												
3 Uptown	575	547.3	133	154.3	45	52.2	72	381.3	118	112.3	117	111.4
8 Near North Side	452	785.7	104	208.7	12	24.1	35	461.3	155	269.4	80	139.1
28 Near West Side	876	1090.9	141	193.2	8	11.0	65	888.2	509	633.9	51	63.5
33 Near South Side	48	766.8	13	239.6	0	0.0	5	598.8	13	207.7	8	127.8
41 Hyde Park	191	529.8	58	188.4	10	32.5	11	208.7	30	83.2	65	180.3
Low Rate Community Areas												
10 Norwood Park	55	182.8	16	60.6	4	15.2	7	190.0	2	6.6	17	56.5
12 Forest Glen	32	217.9	8	62.3	2	15.6	4	217.4	3	20.4	9	61.3
52 East Side	36	214.4	10	67.0	3	20.1	2	107.4	4	23.8	12	71.5
53 West Pullman	43	173.4	11	50.8	5	23.1	3	95.6	6	24.2	12	48.4
55 Hegewisch	13	208.2	5	89.8	2	35.9	0	0.0	1	16.0	4	64.1
64 Clearing	28	218.7	12	100.8	2	16.8	2	223.0	4	31.2	5	39.1
65 West Lawn	43	221.2	16	91.8	0	0.0	1	49.7	5	25.7	11	56.6

TABLE 16
First Admission by Diagnoses for High and Low Rate Mental Hospital Utilization Areas

Community Areas	Total Population #	Rate	Schizo-phrenic #	Rate	Manic-Depressive #	Rate	Senile & Arterio. #	Rate	Alcoholics #	Rate	PP, PN, & PD. #	Rate
High Rate Community Areas												
3 Uptown	189	179.9	28	32.5	17	19.7	8	42.3	43	40.9	66	62.8
8 Near North Side	119	206.8	11	22.1	1	2.0	5	65.2	47	81.6	39	67.7
28 Near West Side	213	265.3	17	23.3	3	4.1	4	54.6	154	191.7	27	33.6
33 Near South Side	13	207.7	3	55.3	0	0.0	0	0.0	6	95.8	3	47.9
41 Hyde Park	71	196.9	15	48.7	3	9.7	0	0.0	9	24.9	38	105.4
Low Rate Community Areas												
10 Norwood Park	27	89.7	9	34.1	2	7.5	1	27.1	0	0.0	12	39.8
12 Forest Glen	19	129.4	4	31.1	1	7.7	2	108.6	2	13.6	6	40.8
52 East Side	17	101.2	4	26.8	1	6.6	0	0.0	2	11.9	8	47.6
53 West Pullman	21	84.7	5	23.1	3	13.8	1	31.8	3	12.0	7	28.2
55 Hegewisch	4	64.1	2	35.9	0	0.0	0	0.0	0	0.0	2	32.0
64 Clearing	17	132.8	7	58.8	1	8.4	1	111.4	1	7.8	4	31.2
65 West Lawn	20	102.9	9	51.6	0	0.0	0	0.0	1	5.1	7	36.0

sclerotic disease are so low as to make interpretation of the rates meaningless. For alcoholism and for PP, PN, and PD the first admission rates parallel the unduplicated rate trend and the high-rate areas for unduplicated admissions generally remains higher. With regard to PP, PN, and PD, Uptown, Near North, and Hyde Park are clearly high, with the rates for Near West and Near South Sides more similar to the range of rates for the low-rate areas.

Table 17 views unduplicated admissions and first admissions by type of institution. The tendency for people generally to utilize state mental hospitals is greater in high-rate areas than in low-rate areas. People from low-rate areas show a tendency to use private institutions and general hospitals more than state mental hospitals. First admissions from high-rate areas are more likely to utilize state mental hospitals than private facilities only in the poor black ghetto areas of the Near West and Near South Sides. The remaining three high-rate areas of Hyde Park, Near North Side, and Uptown are either evenly split or show a preference for the private psychiatric and general hospitals with regard to first admissions. It would appear fairly clear, as one might expect, that the poor go to state mental hospitals and the middle class with hospital insurance go to the private psychiatric or general hospitals.

DISCUSSION AND SUMMARY

a) The Low-Rate Areas

The areas which have a low input into psychiatric inpatient facilities have a quite homogeneous structure. They are mainly lower-middle-class communities. The labor force is made up of a large percentage of blue-collar workers. On the average, people have less than a high school education. The low-rate areas are very stable.

These are areas which are gaining population, but the population gain is white. Most adults are married with young children. There is a high percentage of owner-occupied buildings. The low-rate areas are almost exclusively white. In terms of nativity, there is a large representation of foreign stock (first- and second-generation Americans). These communities tend to have reported low juvenile delinquency rates, low illegitimacy rates, and almost no people on public assistance. When there is need for an in-patient psychiatric service, persons from these areas tend to use private psychiatric and general hospitals rather than public mental hospitals. These areas are low on first hospital admissions as well as unduplicated admissions.

b) The High-Rate Areas

The high-input areas have a number of similarities and also some interesting contrasts among themselves. These areas tend to be heterogeneous in social composition. They tend to be socially and ethnically mixed. Large black populations are to be found in four of the five high-rate areas. The one exception, Uptown, has almost no blacks, but does have a large American Indian and Southern mountain white population. These are areas which are losing total population, but showing gains in black population (except Uptown). These areas tend to be high in indices of poverty. They have large numbers of persons making less than $3,000 per annum. There is a large percentage of unmarried people in these areas. In terms of social problems, these areas have high juvenile delinquency rates, high rates of illegitimacy, and large numbers of people on welfare. People from these areas tend to go to state mental hospitals rather than private psychiatric or general hospitals (as measured by total unduplicated admissions).

Whereas low-rate areas tend to be more like one another on the demographic dimensions reported here, high-rate areas appear to split into a 3-2 grouping. The Near West Side and Near South Side are poverty areas with a large black and/or Spanish-American population. Despite their lower concentration of older persons, they tend to feed large numbers of them into state mental hospitals. They are ghetto areas and poverty is much more pervasive than in the other three high-rate areas. It should be noted, however, that there are a number of other black ghetto areas in Chicago which do not produce an unusual volume of psychiatric casualties. North Lawndale (C.A. 29), Oakland (C.A. 36), and Kenwood (C.A. 39), for example, all produce well below the city average of psychiatric hospital admissions. In fact, the nonwhite utilization rate of mental hospitals for the city as a whole is lower than the non-white representation in the general population. This, coupled with the example of Uptown, should effectively rule out color per se as a special risk factor in mental hospitalization.

The three other high-rate areas, Hyde Park, Near North Side, and Uptown, are not areas where poverty is pervasive and uniform. In these areas there are elements of both the "Gold Coast and the Slum." High-rise apartments are found in these lakefront areas, particularly in Uptown and Near North Side. Two of these areas, Hyde Park and Near North Side, have major universities located within their boundaries. While the Near West Side also contains a major university and a medical center, the professionals who work there do not generally live in the area but commute. This accounts for the higher numbers of college graduates in the Hyde Park and Near North Side areas, higher median incomes, lesser unemployment, and greater numbers of white-collar workers. To a lesser degree, this also holds for Uptown.

Thus, generalization for the high-rate areas is less easy than for the low-rate areas. Low-rate areas are associated with homogeneity, stability, and lower-middle-

TABLE 17
Types of Institutions Used By High and Low Rate Utilization Areas

| | Unduplicated Admissions | | | | | | | | First Admissions | | | | | | | |
| | Total Population | | State Hosp. | | Psych. Unit of Gen. Hospitals | | Private Psych. Hosps. | | Total | | State Hosp. | | Psych. Unit of Gen. Hospitals | | Private Psych. Hosps. |
High Rate Community Areas	#	Rate	#	Rate	#	Rate	#	Rate	#	Rate	#	Rate	#	Rate	#	Rate
3 Uptown	575	547.3	332	316.0	139	132.3	104	98.9	189	179.9	55	52.3	81	77.1	53	50.4
8 Near North Side	452	785.7	328	570.1	86	149.5	38	66.1	119	206.8	49	85.2	53	92.1	17	29.5
28 Near West Side	876	1090.9	833	1037.3	31	38.6	12	14.9	213	265.3	176	219.2	27	33.6	10	12.4
33 Near South Side	48	766.8	42	670.9	2	31.9	4	63.9	13	207.7	7	111.8	2	31.9	4	63.9
41 Hyde Park	191	529.8	101	280.1	72	199.7	18	49.9	71	196.9	11	30.5	48	133.1	12	33.3
Low Rate Community Areas															
10 Norwood Park	55	182.8	12	39.8	18	59.8	25	83.0	27	89.7	2	6.6	13	43.2	12	39.9
12 Forest Glen	32	217.9	9	61.2	16	108.9	7	47.6	19	129.4	3	20.4	9	61.3	7	47.7
52 East Side	36	214.4	12	71.4	12	71.4	12	71.4	17	101.2	2	11.9	4	23.8	11	65.5
53 West Pullman	43	173.4	20	80.6	14	56.4	9	36.2	21	84.7	3	12.1	10	40.3	8	32.3
55 Hegewisch	13	208.2	5	80.0	4	64.0	4	64.0	4	64.0	1	16.0	2	32.0	1	16.0
64 Clearing	28	218.7	7	54.6	16	124.9	5	39.0	17	132.8	1	7.8	12	93.7	4	31.2
65 West Lawn	43	221.2	17	87.4	19	97.7	8	41.1	20	102.9	1	5.1	15	77.2	4	20.0

class value systems and attributes. The low-rate communities not only register a low incidence (as measured by first admissions) of total hospital admissions, but appear to manage their mentally ill better after initial hospitalization, so that readmission is less likely. This attribute is labelled antiextrusion bias. High-rate areas are associated with heterogeneity, instability, rapid social change, and a host of variables associated with poverty and lower-class value systems and attributes. The high-rate areas produce a high incidence of total hospital admissions and appear to lack the capacity to manage their mentally ill after initial hospitalization, so that readmission is more likely. More than this, particularly in socially disorganized areas, such areas appear to foment admissions. This attribute is labelled extrusion bias.

NOTES

1. The Near West Side also contained 19% of all Puerto Ricans and 18% of all Mexicans in Chicago in 1960.

2. One should be reminded of the fact that the reported differences in rates of juvenile delinquency and illegitimacy between lower-class and middle-class areas cannot be accepted as true differences. Middle-class areas keep many instances from the official statistics.

8. ECOLOGICAL ATTRIBUTES OF HIGH AND LOW FIRST ADMISSION RATE AREAS OF CHICAGO

In the previous chapter we were concerned with the ecological attributes of low- and high-rate unduplicated admission areas in Chicago. Now we will examine the characteristics of those communities which exhibit high and
low first admission rates to public, private, and general
hospitals during the study period. A first admission is defined as a person admitted for the first time to a state
mental hospital, a private psychiatric hospital, or the
psychiatric unit of a general hospital with a primary
diagnosis of psychiatric disorder. High first admission
rate community areas are here defined as those with a
rate of 200 or more per year per hundred thousand adult
population. Low first admission rate community areas refer to those with a rate of 45 or less per year per hundred
thousand adult population. These areas are arrayed in
Map 28.

Using these cutting points, we find seven high first admission rate areas. (Henceforth these areas will be abbre-
viated as high and low FARA.) The high FARAs are the
Loop (C.A. 32); the Near North Side, the Near West Side,
and the Near South Side (C.A. 8, 28, and 33, respectively);
one lakefront community on the north, Rogers Park

123

Map 28—High and low first admission rate areas

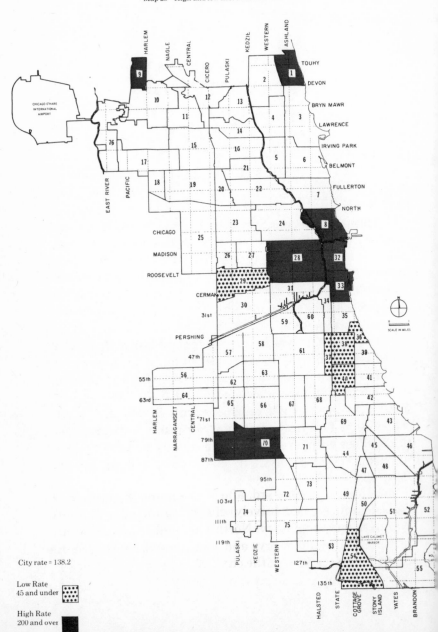

City rate = 138.2

Low Rate
45 and under

High Rate
200 and over

(C.A. 1); and two semisuburban communities, Edison Park in the far northwest (C.A. 9) and Ashburn in the far southwest (C.A. 70). It was decided to exclude the Loop from further analysis, as we did in the analysis of high unduplicated admission rate areas. The reasons were the same. The Loop is a highly atypical area with a small resident population and a very high rate of first admission (1355/100,000 adult population), a rate some 10 times the citywide average of 138/100,000 adult population.

The Loop and its three adjacent areas to the north, west, and south stand out clearly as high FARAs of the city. These four areas also stood out clearly as the highest unduplicated admission areas of the city. This is an important finding on two counts. These are the same areas which showed the highest rates of first admissions in Faris and Dunham's study some thirty years prior and it now emerges that these areas not only produce a high over-all psychiatric casualty rate, but also contribute disproportionately to the count of persons being initially hospitalized for a psychiatric disorder. Rogers Park, to a lesser degree, exhibits both these attributes, being a high FARA and having a higher than average unduplicated admission rate (459/100,000). The two remaining high FARAs, Edison Park and Ashburn, lie on the outlying perimeter of the city and both are relatively low in unduplicated admissions, though neither falls into the category of low unduplicated admission areas as defined in the previous chapter (225/100,000 or less).

The six low FARAs are the areas of Oakland, Fuller Park, Grand Boulevard, and Washington Park (C.A. 36, 37, 38 and 40, respectively) clustering in the near southeastern part of the city; North Lawndale (C.A. 29) on the west central periphery; and Riverdale (C.A. 54) on the southern perimeter of the city.

TABLE 18
Sex, Race, Age, and Growth Characteristics
of High and Low First Admission Rate Areas in 1960

C.A.	Population	Male No.	%	Female No.	%	White No.	%	Black No.	%	% 18 and Under	% 65 and Over	Total Population	Black Population
High First Admissions Areas, White													
1 Rogers Park	56,888	25,755	45.3	31,133	54.7	56,503	99.3	57	—	21.0	14.2	- 8.6	—
9 Edison Park	12,568	6,013	47.8	6,555	52.2	12,565	99.9	—	—	34.1	9.7	—	—
70 Ashburn	38,638	19,188	49.7	19,450	50.3	38,604	99.9	1	—	43.4	3.9	417.1	—
High First Admissions Areas, Black													
8 Near North Side	75,509	38,031	50.4	37,478	49.6	50,569	67.0	23,114	30.6	26.2	10.2	-15.3	29.8
28 Near West Side	126,610	67,056	53.0	59,554	47.0	57,676	45.6	68,146	53.8	40.5	5.8	-21.0	4.0
33 Near South Side	10,350	5,248	50.7	5,102	49.3	2,354	22.7	7,942	76.7	42.9	8.1	- 8.5	1.4
Low First Admission Areas													
29 North Lawndale	124,937	60,054	48.1	64,883	51.9	10,792	8.6	113,827	91.1	46.4	3.3	24.3	765.9
36 Oakland	24,378	11,399	46.8	12,979	53.2	311	1.3	23,955	98.3	46.3	4.7	- 0.4	26.6
37 Fuller Park	12,181	5,900	48.4	6,281	51.6	476	3.9	11,692	95.9	44.7	4.4	-29.1	36.8
38 Grand Boulevard	80,036	38,155	47.7	41,881	52.3	398	0.5	79,537	99.4	30.9	9.4	-30.1	-29.8
40 Washington Park	43,690	20,977	48.0	22,713	52.0	332	0.8	43,310	99.1	25.7	9.7	-23.2	-22.9
54 Riverdale	11,448	5,346	46.7	6,102	53.3	1,127	9.8	10,306	90.0	63.0	2.7	16.9	25.0

ECOLOGICAL COMPARISON
OF HIGH AND
LOW FARAs

Table 18 arrays the data on sex, race, age, and community growth characteristics for the six high and six low FARAs. The sex distribution for high and low FARAs is approximately equal. The low FARAs are all preponderantly black, ranging from Riverdale (90%) to Grand Boulevard (99.4%). The high FARAs break into two groups of three on the color dimension. Rogers Park, Edison Park, and Ashburn have practically no black population (all under 1%). The Near North, Near West, and Near South Sides show substantial black population (30.6%, 53.8% and 76.7%, respectively), all above the reported 1960 citywide average of 23% black population. One should note the fact that these three areas are quite racially and ethnically mixed. In this and subsequent breakdowns, the white high FARAs and the predominantly black high FARAs will be separately grouped for ease of analysis.

The age characteristics of the high and low FARAs are totally mixed, both with regard to percentage of persons over 65 and persons under 18. Also, no pattern is discernible with regard to population growth characteristics.

Nativity characteristics are arrayed in Table 19. There is a clear trend for the high FARAs to have substantially higher numbers of foreign born and native born with foreign parentage. The white high FARAs have substantially more second-generation Americans than the black high FARAs which in turn have a substantially higher percentage of second-generation Americans than the low FARAs. Low FARAs are composed predominantly of native born with native parentage (95.6%-99.2% for the six low FARAs). This is a reversal of the finding reported in the previous chapter on unduplicated admissions, where low-rate areas were predominantly composed of second-generation Americans. In both cases nativity is an expression of race since black people are not likely to have foreign parents or themselves be immigrants.

Table 20 deals with marital status. White high FARAs have substantially the same percentage of single persons as the low FARAs. It is the three black high FARAs which show a substantial elevation of percentage single persons over the other nine areas. This pattern is reversed for percent married. For separated and divorced persons, the white high FARAs show a very low percent

TABLE 19
Nativity Percentages of High and Low
First Admission Rate Areas in 1960

High First Admission Areas, White		Percentages		
C.A:	Total	Foreign Born	Native: Foreign or Mixed Parentage	Native: Native Parentage
1 Rogers Park	100.0	17.7	30.7	51.6
9 Edison Park	100.0	8.0	30.4	61.6
70 Ashburn	100.0	6.2	27.9	65.9
High First Admission Areas, Black				
8 Near North Side	100.0	7.7	12.6	79.7
28 Near West Side	100.0	7.5	10.5	82.0
33 Near South Side	100.0	3.1	3.1	93.8
Low First Admisson Areas				
29 North Lawndale	100.0	1.8	2.6	95.6
36 Oakland	100.0	0.4	0.4	99.2
37 Fuller Park	100.0	1.0	1.5	97.5
38 Grand Boulevard	100.0	0.3	0.7	99.0
40 Washington	100.0	0.5	0.6	98.9
54 Riverdale	100.0	1.1	2.6	96.3

TABLE 20

Marital Status Percentages by Sex for High and Low First Admission Rate Areas in 1960

C.A.	Total Percentages					Female Percentages					Male Percentages				
	Sing.	Marr.	Sep.	Wid.	Div.	Sing.	Marr.	Sep.	Wid.	Div.	Sing.	Marr.	Sep.	Wid.	Div.
High First Admission Areas-White															
1 Rogers Park	22.9	61.6	1.2	11.5	4.0	22.3	55.5	1.3	17.1	5.1	23.6	69.4	1.0	4.4	2.6
9 Edison Park	19.9	70.4	0.5	8.3	1.3	19.5	66.4	0.7	12.3	1.8	20.4	75.0	0.4	3.8	0.8
70 Ashburn	16.7	69.6	0.4	7.5	1.4	15.4	75.3	0.6	8.0	1.3	18.1	79.0	0.3	2.2	0.7
High First Admission Areas-Black															
8 Near North Side	39.4	45.0	4.6	9.5	6.2	34.9	44.8	5.1	13.9	6.4	43.9	45.0	4.1	5.1	6.0
28 Near West Side	31.7	55.6	8.9	8.4	4.3	23.7	60.6	10.4	11.9	3.8	38.4	51.4	7.7	5.5	4.7
33 Near South Side	28.2	54.3	12.4	12.3	5.1	22.3	57.5	14.9	15.2	5.0	33.7	51.4	10.1	9.7	5.2
Low First Admission Areas															
29 North Lawndale	23.6	66.1	9.3	7.1	3.2	20.6	65.4	12.1	10.1	3.9	27.1	66.8	6.1	3.7	2.4
36 Oakland	22.7	62.1	13.8	10.6	4.6	19.1	60.7	17.0	14.6	5.6	27.2	63.8	9.9	5.6	3.4
37 Fuller Park	24.4	63.5	9.4	8.6	3.5	21.1	62.7	10.8	12.5	3.7	28.0	64.5	7.7	4.2	3.3
38 Grand Boulevard	20.6	58.3	13.1	15.8	5.3	16.6	56.6	14.1	20.9	5.9	25.2	60.2	12.0	10.0	4.6
40 Washington Park	19.6	59.8	12.5	13.9	6.7	15.6	58.3	13.2	18.8	7.3	24.0	61.6	11.8	8.4	6.0
54 Riverdale	28.8	61.2	9.5	6.7	3.4	23.7	61.2	16.0	9.8	5.3	35.6	61.2	0.9	2.5	0.7

129

TABLE 21
Education, Employment, and Family Income Characteristics of High and Low First Admission Rate Areas in 1960

C.A.	Education		Percent of all workers in mfg.	Employment		Family Income		
	Median School Year Comp. (1959)	Percent with 4 or more years College		Percent of all males in white-coll. occup.	Percent of Labor Force Unemployed	Median Family Income	Percent with Income Under $3,000	Percent With Income Over $10,000
High First Admission Areas, White								
1 Rogers Park	12.2	14.3	22.2	66.2	2.3	7,465	9.8	27.4
9 Edison Park	12.1	9.0	32.7	53.4	2.1	9,185	5.3	42.2
70 Ashburn	12.1	6.2	32.0	42.2	1.6	8,382	2.6	29.6
High First Admission Areas, Black								
8 Near North Side	12.0	17.9	17.0	55.3	5.8	5,532	24.2	27.4
28 Near West Side	8.3	3.5	29.3	21.5	11.6	3,984	36.8	5.3
33 Near South Side	8.6	2.9	25.2	20.5	14.5	3,280	46.0	5.0
Low First Admission Areas								
29 North Lawndale	8.7	1.5	36.1	16.1	10.0	4,981	24.8	8.7
36 Oakland	8.8	1.4	25.7	16.7	15.0	3,412	44.8	2.8
37 Fuller Park	8.5	0.9	34.7	14.8	12.1	4,547	28.1	7.3
38 Grand Boulevard	8.7	2.3	22.9	16.9	12.3	4,329	32.6	5.6
40 Washington Park	9.0	2.7	25.2	20.3	11.0	4,806	25.6	7.2
54 Riverdale	10.1	1.9	35.6	18.2	16.1	3,261	46.8	4.6

compared to the predominantly black areas whether they are high or low FARAs. This pattern is elaborated by sex breakdown. Percent female separated and divorced is lower for the three white high FARAs compared to the predominantly black areas. For males, the three black high FARAs are substantially higher in percent single than the remaining nine areas. The percentage of married males for the three white high FARAs is higher than in the low FARAs, whose figures are in turn higher than those in the three predominantly black high FARAs. The marital status variable appears to relate most strongly to race and poverty, with more evidence of isolated individuals and broken families in the black high FARAs.

The breakdown of education, employment, and income characteristics as arrayed in Table 21 is practically uniform in its differentiation of predominantly black from white areas regardless of first admission rate characteristics. White areas have higher levels of education, greater numbers of white-collar workers, lower rates of unemployment, higher median incomes, fewer persons in abject poverty, and more persons living in relative affluence than black areas. The only variable considered in Table 21 which does not show a clear black-white differentiation is the percentage of blue-collar workers. It should be noted that the Near North Side (C.A. 8) is more nearly like the all-white areas. While this area is one-third black, the area also has a substantial white population, many of whom are quite affluent. This area also houses a major university complex and medical center.

Table 22 reports differences in housing characteristics between the high and low FARAs. There is a clear tendency for high FARAs to have more new houses than low FARAs. Owner-occupied homes predominate only in the semisuburban areas of Edison Park and Ashburn which are high FARAs; otherwise rates of home owner-

TABLE 22

Housing Characteristics of High and Low First Admission Rate Areas in 1960

C.A.	Percent Built 1950 or Later	Percent Owner Occupied	Percent Substandard Housing	Percent more than one person per room	Percent with Med. value owner units in one unit structures	Median number of rooms	Median Gross Rent, Renter units
High First Admission Areas, White							
1 Rogers Park	6.3	11.3	2.6	4.2	20,300	3.9	110
9 Edison Park	41.8	83.1	0.6	5.9	22,400	5.3	113
70 Ashburn	87.2	95.1	0.2	12.3	19,700	5.2	114
High First Admission Areas, Black							
8 Near North Side	14.5	6.0	34.8	12.8	25,000+	2.3	82
28 Near West Side	10.0	9.6	44.4	28.9	12,400	3.6	66
33 Near South Side	22.3	1.6	52.8	30.1	—	2.3	64
Low First Admission Areas							
29 North Lawndale	1.1	17.9	14.0	35.0	15,200	4.3	97
36 Oakland	4.5	5.9	44.6	38.6	16,300	2.6	72
37 Fuller Park	1.7	28.4	24.9	31.1	12,800	4.6	92
38 Grand Boulevard	1.6	7.6	43.9	22.1	17,000	3.3	79
40 Washington Park	0.5	6.9	37.0	18.2	16,300	3.5	85
54 Riverdale	18.5	11.2	1.6	48.2	10,800	4.5	66

Housing Data

ship are roughly similar among the remaining areas. Substandard housing runs high in black areas with the notable exception of Riverdale, a low FARA. Riverdale, together with the three white high FARAs of Rogers Park, Edison Park, and Ashburn, has a negligible rate of substandard housing. The black-white differential continues on the population density measure, but there is some tendency for low FARAs to have a higher percentage of dwellings with more than one person per room. Dwelling size in the three black high FARAs tends to be smaller than in the other nine areas. Median value of dwellings is higher in the white than in the black areas and there is a tendency for high FARAs to have higher-value dwellings. Rents in the black areas are lower than in the white areas with no obvious relation over-all to rates of first admissions.

Table 23 presents data on juvenile delinquency, illegitimate births, and public assistance. Here again, on all three indices the black-white differentiation appears to override any general variation between high and low FARAs. The three white high FARAs have very low rates of reported juvenile delinquency, illegitimate pregnancy, and welfare recipients. One must, of course, accept the statistics on delinquency and pregnancy with caution since there is unquestionably under-reporting on these variables from the white areas. The rates for these three social disorganization indices are uniformly high for the black areas with the exception of Riverdale which reports somewhat lower rates of juvenile delinquency and illegitimate pregnancy than the other black areas, but still far in excess of the white areas.

Table 24 presents data on psychiatric diagnosis for first admissions. When total first admissions are broken down by diagnosis, the numbers admitted by community areas are so small that meaningful comparisons are difficult to make. Rates of first admissions in every diagnostic category except senile and arteriosclerotic disease are

TABLE 23
Selected Social Problem Indicators of High and Low First Admission Rate Areas

C.A.	No. of Males brought before Family Court of Cook County on deling. petitions 1958-61		Illegitimate Births (1962)		Public Assistance (1962)	
		Rate/100 Boys 12-16		Percent of		Recipients/ 100 popula-
	Number	yrs.	Number	Live Births	Total	tion
High First Admission Areas, White						
1 Rogers Park	15	1.1	17	2.1	530	0.9
9 Edison Park	6	1.0	1	0.8	40	0.3
70 Ashburn	12	0.8	4	1.3	40	0.1
High First Admission Areas, Black						
8 Near North Side	108	6.2	611	29.7	12,680	16.8
28 Near West Side	288	6.1	1,021	25.8	31,240	24.7
33 Near South Side	34	8.5	95	36.4	3,410	32.9
Low First Admission Areas						
29 North Lawndale	320	7.0	1,563	33.0	32,270	25.8
36 Oakland	50	5.8	324	37.7	10,090	41.4
37 Fuller Park	28	5.6	95	29.1	2,250	18.5
38 Grand Boulevard	176	7.6	840	32.6	22,910	28.6
40 Washington Park	59	5.2	280	26.9	7,940	18.2
54 Riverdale	22	2.9	64	20.8	4,530	39.6

134

TABLE 24
Number and Rate of First Admissions to 44 Public and Private Mental Hospitals by Diagnosis for High and Low First Admission Rate Areas from July 1, 1960 to June 30, 1961

C.A.	Total People		Schizophrenic		Manic-Depressive Psychosis		Senile and Arteriosclerotic		Alcoholic		P.P., P.N., and P.D.	
	No.	Rate	No.	Rate	No.	Rate	No.	Rate	No.	Rate	No.	Rate
High First Admission Areas, White												
1 Rogers Park	97	208.2	16	41.5	11	28.5	5	62.1	5	10.7	47	100.9
9 Edison Park	18	202.5	3	39.1	0	0.0	2	163.3	0	0.0	10	112.5
70 Ashburn	29	217.2	5	42.2	3	25.3	1	66.4	1	7.4	17	-127.3
High First Admission Areas, Black												
8 Near North Side	119	206.8	11	22.1	1	2.0	5	65.2	47	81.6	39	67.7
28 Near West Side	213	265.3	16	21.9	3	4.1	4	54.7	154	191.8	27	33.6
33 Near South Side	13	207.7	3	55.3	0	0.0	0	0.0	6	95.8	3	47.9
Low First Admission Areas												
29 North Lawndale	27	37.3	8	11.7	1	1.5	6	144.9	3	4.1	7	9.7
36 Oakland	6	42.9	2	15.6	0	0.0	2	173.6	1	7.1	1	7.1
37 Fuller Park	2	27.4	1	14.8	0	0.0	0	0.0	0	0.0	1	13.7
38 Grand Boulevard	22	38.0	5	9.9	0	0.0	1	13.3	6	10.4	7	12.1
40 Washington Park	11	32.6	2	6.8	0	0.0	1	23.7	0	0.0	5	14.8
54 Riverdale	2	40.5	0	0.0	1	21.6	0	0.0	0	0.0	1	20.2

TABLE 25

Number and Rate of Unduplicated Admissions to 44 Public and Private Mental Hospitals by Diagnosis for High and Low First Admission Rate Areas from July 1, 1960 to June 30, 1961

C.A.	Total People		Schizo-phrenic		Manic-Depressive Psychosis		Senile and Arterio-sclerotic		Alcoholic		P.P., P.N., and P.D.	
	No.	Rate	No.	Rate	No.	Rate	No.	Rate	No.	Rate	No.	Rate
High First Admission Areas, White												
1 Rogers Park	214	459.3	51	132.3	20	51.9	17	211.1	12	25.8	75	161.0
9 Edison Park	24	270.0	4	52.2	0	0.0	4	326.5	1	11.3	11	123.8
70 Ashburn	44	329.6	12	101.3	3	25.3	3	199.2	3	22.5	19	142.3
High First Admission Areas, Black												
8 Near North Side	452	785.7	104	208.7	12	24.1	35	461.3	155	269.4	80	139.1
28 Near West Side	876	1090.9	141	193.2	8	11.0	65	888.2	509	633.9	51	63.5
33 Near South Side	48	766.8	13	239.6	0	0.0	5	598.8	13	207.7	8	127.8
Low First Admission Areas												
29 North Lawndale	213	294.2	92	134.8	3	4.4	19	458.9	34	47.0	18	24.9
36 Oakland	60	428.7	23	179.1	0	0.0	10	868.1	13	92.9	5	35.7
37 Fuller Park	23	314.9	9	132.8	1	14.8	3	566.0	4	54.8	1	13.7
38 Grand Boulevard	228	393.4	77	152.6	4	7.9	39	520.6	38	65.6	18	31.1
40 Washington Park	143	423.7	46	155.8	2	6.8	20	473.3	28	83.0	15	44.4
54 Riverdale	19	384.5	9	194.2	1	21.6	1	325.7	0	0.0	3	60.7

clearly higher in the high FARAs. The preponderant diagnoses of patients from high FARAs are alcoholism and PP, PN, and PD. That data also suggests that the diagnoses of manic-depressive psychosis and PP, PN, and PD disorders are more liberally applied to whites than to blacks.

Table 25 records unduplicated admissions for various psychiatric disorders emanating from the high and low FARAs. Low FARAs for all diagnoses are also low in unduplicated admissions for all diagnoses. However, white high FARAs record relatively low unduplicated admissions, while black high FARAs record very high unduplicated admissions. The unduplicated admission rate for schizophrenia for the black high FARAs is generally somewhat higher than for the low FARAs. The small numbers of patients diagnosed as manic-depressive do not allow meaningful comparison. For black areas, rates of unduplicated admissions for senile and arteriosclerotic disease are higher than for white areas. For black high FARAs, alcoholic unduplicated admissions are very high, much higher than for either white high FARAs or low FARAs. PP, PN, and PD rates for high FARAs are uniformly higher than for low FARAs and tend to be higher in the white FARAs than in the black high FARAs.

Table 26 reports first admissions and unduplicated admissions to state mental hospitals, private mental hospitals, and general hospitals. With regard to first admissions to state mental hospitals, the three black high FARAs are clearly higher than the low FARAs. The three white FARAs are not substantially different from the six low FARAs on state hospital first admissions. With regard to psychiatric units of general hospitals, the three white high FARAs are higher than the three black high FARAs which in turn are higher than the six low FARAs. With regard to private psychiatric hospitals, the

TABLE 26

Number and Rate per 100,000 of People Admitted to 44 Public and Private Mental Hospitals by Type of Institution for High and Low First Admission Rate Areas from July 1, 1960 to June 30, 1961

C.A.	First Admissions								Unduplicated Admissions							
	Total		State Hospitals		Psych. Units of Gen. Hosp.		Private Psych. Hosps.		Total		State Hospitals		Psych. Units of Gen. Hosp.		Private Psych. Hosp.	
	No.	Rate	No.	Rate	No.	Rate	No.	Rate	No.	Rate	No.	Rate	No.	Rate	No.	Rate
High First Admission Areas, White																
1 Rogers Park	97	208.2	5	10.7	59	126.6	33	70.8	214	459.3	64	137.4	91	195.3	59	126.6
9 Edison Park	18	202.5	2	22.5	9	101.3	7	78.8	24	270.0	4	45.0	10	112.5	10	112.5
70 Ashburn	29	217.2	1	7.5	25	187.3	3	22.5	44	329.6	7	52.4	32	239.7	4	30.0
High First Admission Areas-Black																
8 Near North Side	119	206.8	49	85.2	53	92.1	17	29.5	452	785.7	328	570.1	86	149.5	38	66.1
28 Near West Side	213	265.3	176	219.2	27	33.6	10	12.4	876	1090.9	833	1037.4	31	38.6	12	14.9
33 Near South Side	13	207.7	7	111.8	2	31.9	4	63.9	48	766.8	42	670.9	2	31.9	4	68.9
Low First Admission Areas																
29 North Lawndale	27	37.3	8	11.0	11	15.2	8	11.0	213	294.2	189	261.0	15	20.7	9	12.4
36 Oakland	6	42.9	3	21.4	2	14.3	1	7.1	60	428.7	57	407.3	2	14.3	1	7.1
37 Fuller Park	2	27.4	1	13.7	0	0.0	1	13.7	23	314.9	20	273.8	1	13.7	2	27.4
38 Grand Boulevard	22	38.0	15	25.9	5	8.6	2	3.5	228	393.4	220	379.6	6	10.4	2	3.5
40 Washington Park	11	32.6	6	17.8	4	11.9	1	3.0	143	423.7	136	402.9	5	14.8	2	5.9
54 Riverdale	2	40.5	2	40.5	0	0.0	0	0.0	19	384.5	19	384.5	0	0.0	0	0.0

high FARAs are clearly higher than the low FARAs, but again the more meaningful comparison is the white versus the black areas; the white areas are significant users of private psychiatric hospitals while the black ʾreas are only very occasional users.

When one examines unduplicated admissions from high and low FARAs into state mental hospitals, the three white high FARAs are clearly low. The three black high FARAs are very high and the six low FARAs fall in between. The opposite pattern is true for general hospitals where the three white high FARAs are higher than the three black high FARAs which in turn are higher than the low FARAs. With regard to private psychiatric hospitals, the high FARAs are much higher in unduplicated admissions than the low FARAs with the white areas using the private psychiatric hospitals substantially and the black areas hardly at all.

DISCUSSION

There are several major findings in the data presented in this chapter. It turns out that of the seven highest FARAs of the city, four are also found in the list of the six highest unduplicated admission areas. These are the Loop, the Near North, the Near West, and the Near South Sides (C.A. 32, 8, 28, and 33 respectively). This is a finding which is most provocative. These four areas constitute the central heart of the city and are the same areas reported by Faris and Dunham as the highest first admissions rate areas some thirty years prior. That these areas are highest in both first admissions and unduplicated admissions means that not only are these areas highly productive of psychiatric casualties generally, but they also show a high incidence of psychiatric disorder of all kinds. The Near North, Near West, and Near South Sides, which have significant black as well as Spanish-

American populations, are high on poverty indices and indices of social disorganization. The remaining three high FARAs, Rogers Park, Edison Park, and Ashburn (C.A. 1, 9, and 70 respectively), are white areas located at the periphery of the city. Racially, socially, and economically, they differ in the extreme from the central-city high FARAs.

The six low FARAs are all black areas (over 90%). This is a complete reversal of the character of the seven lowest rate unduplicated admission areas reported in the previous chapter which were all over 99% white. Five of these six low FARAs may be classified as inner city ghetto areas. These are North Lawndale, Oakland, Fuller Park, Grand Boulevard, and Washington Park (C.A. 29, 36, 37, 38, and 40 respectively). Four of these areas (C.A. 36, 37, 38, and 40) are contiguous and in common with C.A. 29 are all close to the city center, and in fact adjoin the high-rate central city areas on the west and south (see Map 28). All fall at or below the citywide unduplicated admission rate of 429/100,000 adult population.

Herein lies the first of two significant differences with the findings of Faris and Dunham. While the central city areas are indeed high FARAs, as was found previously by those authors, the rates of first admissions do not drop off in any uniform way as we proceed from the city center to the periphery. In fact, the lowest FARAs in the present study are, with only one exception, inner city ghetto areas which adjoin the city center. On the city periphery are found three of the high FARAs and one low FARA. The second significant difference with the Faris and Dunham findings has been already mentioned in the previous chapter and this is the apparently random distribution of schizophrenic first admissions over the entire map of the city. This latter conclusion is weakened by the fact that the entire number of first admission schizophrenics was 634 during the study period. When this number is apportioned among 75 community areas, the rate for any given area may be assumed to be fairly unreliable.

There are some central problems in the interpretation of the data reported in this chapter and the last. Why are some predominantly black areas highly productive of psychiatric casualties while other black areas, often adjacent, are not? What communalities, if any, exist between black areas and white areas which share the common characteristic of producing a high volume of psychiatric casualties? Why are the six lowest FARAs 90% or more black while the seven lowest unduplicated admission areas 99% or more white?

The following considerations which bear on the above questions are suggested by our data:

1. *The Changing Neighborhood.*   The seven all-white low unduplicated admission rate areas and the six black low FARAs are racially stable areas. The six high unduplicated admission rate areas and the seven high FARAs (four areas are actually in both groups) are in the main undergoing significant change. This change is apparent in influx and outflux of people, transiency, significant urban renewal, changes in racial and ethnic composition, and high degrees of social disorganization which result in less cohesive communal and family structure. It is a fact that the more rapidly changing parts of the city are located centrally and that the neighborhoods on the periphery of the city are less prone to rapid change. The end product of this process will be all black or Spanish-American impoverished inner cities and white middle class suburbs, a conclusion which is being widely predicted by demographers.

2. *Racial Balance.*   Independent of the consideration of change is the issue of racial and ethnic proportions. It would appear that persons living in racially and ethnical-

ly mixed areas are at higher risk of hospitalization for mental illness than persons living in racially homogeneous areas. In the four areas which register both the highest rate of first admissions and the highest rate of unduplicated admissions (C.A. 32, 8, 28, and 33), the percent black population is 10.4, 30.6, 53.8, and 76.7 respectively. In addition, some of these areas contain significant numbers of Spanish-Americans as well as white population. The high unduplicated admission areas of Hyde Park and Uptown (C.A. 41 and 3) are quite mixed racially and ethnically. Hyde Park has a 37.7% black population with the remainder mainly white. Uptown has substantial representation of southern mountain whites, Japanese-Americans, and American Indians. These areas contrast with the seven low rate unduplicated admission areas which are 99%+ white and the six low FARAs which are 90% + black.

3. *Poverty.* While indices of poverty are clearly and positively correlated with rate of unduplicated admissions, these indices are not so clearly related to rates of first admission. This is interpreted to mean that poverty per se is not related to the production of new cases of psychiatric disorder (incidence) but is related to the total pool of cases available at any given time (prevalence). Some relatively affluent areas such as Edison Park and Ashburn produce high rates of new psychiatric cases as do the poor areas of the Near West and Near South Sides. However, cases admitted from the more affluent areas are less likely to be readmitted after discharge than cases admitted from poor areas. Patients entering a mental hospital for the first time who have some means will enter a general hospital or private psychiatric hospital and will receive better treatment than is available in a public hospital and better aftercare upon discharge. These factors, and others, will conspire to lower the undu-

plicated admission rate from a middle-class area, whereas the first admission rates may be comparable to a lower-class area.

4. *Jail or Hospital?* It is also possible that deviant behavior, particularly aggressive antisocial behavior, is labelled differently and the persons exhibiting the behavior handled differently when it occurs in the poor inner city area as compared with a semisuburban more affluent community. The police are conditioned to react differently to a poor black person than to an affluent white person exhibiting the same behavior. Also the community setting will tend to elicit different responses; in a slum objective danger to the policeman will be greater than in a middle class neighborhood. A poor black person seen acting out aggressively is more likely to be arrested and charged and his extrusion route out of the community is likely to be to prison. The affluent white person seen in the same circumstances may be brought to a mental health facility and his extrusion route is likely to be via the mental hospital. We can present no data to directly support this contention, but it is a fact that Chicago mental hospital admissions are more often white in proportion to the numbers of whites in the population and Chicago prison admissions are more often black in proportion to their numbers in the population.

THE CONCEPT OF
EXTRUSION AND
ANTIEXTRUSION BIAS

It would appear that communities respond differently to behavioral symptoms of severe psychiatric disorder. Certain communities foment admissions to a mental hospital when confronted with peculiar or offensive deviant behavior. We do not believe that the incidence of such behavior varies very much from community to community in Chicago or at different points in time in a given community. Numbers of persons first admitted to public mental hospitals in Illinois have remained relatively constant during the period 1960-1970, although unduplicated admissions have increased about 25% (Levy, 1971).

A person exhibiting symptoms of a severe mental disorder who is without means, who has no immediate family, who is marginally employed or unemployed, and who lives in a community without cohesive social structure is a prime candidate for admission to a public mental hospital. If, in addition, he is black, he may also be a likely candidate for admission into our penal system. In either case, the community in which he resides has a clear extrusion bias. There is very little to hinder and much to facilitate extrusion of the mentally-ill person into a mental hospital or other extracommunity holding facility such as a nursing home, or prison, or an institution for the retarded.

A person developing a serious nervous disorder who resides in a socially cohesive community where he has a family, a job, membership in various social, religious, business, or professional organizations and within which frameworks he is far from anonymous will not be extruded from the community as easily or as quickly. Money and social status are important factors in securing out-patient treatment for a mental disorder. Thus we may expect that affluent persons will receive out-patient care as an alternative to hospitalization more often than the poor. When hospitalization occurs, the person with means and middle-class social credentials will fare better in terms of quality of treatment than the lower-class person and thus stand a better chance of improvement and decreased probability of subsequent readmissions.

Another factor which affects the extrusion bias of a community is its attitude towards psychiatry. Psychiatry has traditionally appealed to an upper-middle-class privileged clientele. Blue-collar workers often react with suspicion and hostility to "headshrinkers" and one may suppose that the low rate of unduplicated admissions from blue-collar communities reflects in part this feeling. The lower-middle-class person with a nervous disorder may look to and receive care from his family doctor who will either not hospitalize him or do so in a general hospital without making a psychiatric diagnosis.

The higher rates of use of mental hospitals by both lower-class and upper-middle-class communities may reflect a lack of choice for the lower-class community residents and a positive preference by the upper-middle-class community resident. In communities such as Hyde Park or the Near North Side, where a professional upper-middle-class community, mainly peripheral to a university, and a lower-class community, mainly black, coexist, high admission rates may be contributed to by both sectors.

In brief, the extrusion bias of a community is determined by a collection of community traits, institutions, and prevalent communal beliefs and attitudes towards mental illness and its treatment which either foment or hinder mental hospital admissions or other forms of egress for its deviants from the community. The concept is of some theoretical importance, because believing as we do that the incidence of major mental disorder does not vary greatly from place to place or from time to time, what must explain observed differential rates of hospital admission is the manner in which the community deals with mental illness.

9. MAJOR FINDINGS AND CONCLUDING OBSERVATIONS

Analysis of characteristics of persons admitted to inpatient psychiatric facilities from the city of Chicago during a one-year period and analysis of their communities of residence prior to hospitalization yielded the following results:

1. More men than women were admitted—a reversal of the sex distribution in the Chicago population.

2. Women showed a more stable pattern of hospitalization regardless of place of residence while male admissions tended to come from the lower socio-economic areas.

3. Blacks utilize mental hospitals less in proportion to their representation in the population than whites.

4. Black admissions are highest in those areas with the smallest percentage of black residents.

5. Blacks receive a disproportionate share of the diagnosis schizophrenia.

6. White males receive a disproportionate share of the alcoholic diagnosis.

7. White females are diagnosed predominantly as schizophrenic or psychoneurotic.

8. Women, regardless of race, tend to be diagnosed schizophrenic to a greater extent than men.

9. Persons under 25 are under represented and persons over 65 are over represented in the patient population studied compared to their representation in the Chicago population.

10. Geriatric admissions are low in areas which are white, lower-middle-class communities with a large percentage of foreign stock.

11. The patient population showed proportionately more single, widowed, separated, and divorced persons than the population at large.

12. Married persons utilized mental hospitals less than persons not married.

13. Never-married persons show higher mental hospital utilization than persons who have been widowed, divorced, or separated.

14. Schizophrenia, diseases of the senium, and alcoholism are found to be associated with communities which are characterized by social instability and poverty.

15. The data on admissions for schizophrenia and diseases of the senium appear to support a drift or social selection phenomenon in that first admissions for these diagnoses tend to come from more affluent communities while readmissions tend to emanate from poorer communities.

16. Patients carrying the diagnoses of psychophysiologic, psychoneurotic, and personality disorder and persons carrying the diagnosis of manic-depressive psychosis tend to come from higher socio-economic areas.

17. Schizophrenic first admissions tend to be distributed in a random fashion over the city while readmissions predominate in the communities comprising the city center and along the lakeshore.

18. Manic-depressive first admissions and readmissions tend to come from middle-class areas.

19. Alcoholic first admissions and readmissions are both concentrated in the city-center areas.

20. Senile first admissions come from all over the city, but one cluster of high first admission rate areas is found in the city center. Senile readmissions are concentrated in the city center.

21. Psychophysiologic, psychoneurotic, and personality disorder first admissions and readmissions show a scattering throughout the city. First admission high rate areas are primarily middle class or with a strong middle-class component. High readmission areas are represented by both lower and middle class areas.

22. A majority of persons admitted to in-patient psychiatric facilities during the study period went to state mental hospitals. A majority of the first admissions, however, went to private mental hospitals or general hospitals.

23. Whether one uses a public or private facility appears to be a function of social class.

24. Low unduplicated admission rate areas have associated characteristics of homogeneity, stability, and lower-middle-class values and attributes.

25. High unduplicated admission rate areas have associated characteristics of heterogeneity, instability, rapid social change, poverty, and lower-class value systems and attributes.

26. Low first admission rate areas are generally racially homogeneous and stable.

27. High first admission rate areas are generally heterogeneous and unstable.

28. High first admission rate areas are in the main undergoing significant social change reflected in influx and outflux of people, transiency, significant urban renewal, changes in racial and ethnic composition, and high degrees of social disorganization manifested in less cohesive communal and familial structure.

CONCLUDING OBSERVATIONS

a) Age

This study is primarily concerned with adult psychiatric admissions, not by design but by circumstance. Few children under 15 are admitted into the mental hospital system. This is largely due to the absence of facilities for receiving them.

Old persons are at specially high risk of mental hospitalization largely because of social dislocation. Our attitude towards aging persons in America is barbaric and one index of this attitude is the funneling of aging persons into warehouses of one sort or another to live out the final years of their lives. If an old person is fortunate enough to have accumulated means during his working years, then to the extent that his health and stamina are unimpaired, and to the degree that he is related to a social subculture which has a responsible attitude towards its senior members, he may be able to maintain his autonomy and some semblance of a human existence.

b) Sex

That male admissions exceed female admissions is a curiosity. That male admissions tend to come from lower socio-economic areas while female admissions show a more uniform pattern of residence prior to hospitalization is of greater interest. This finding is believed to be another of the several which we observed which conformed to the postulation of a drift phenomenon. Disabling psychiatric illness for a man appears to mean social mobility downwards. The family gets more and more financially pressed as the breadwinner becomes less able to work. With women, on the other hand, this is seldom the case. The female is as yet not the determiner of the family's social class. If the female is psychiatrically disabled, bills for her care may mount, but this will not affect her husband's earning capacity, and hence their social class or neighborhood of residence. This argument is strengthened by the finding in our data that women are diagnosed schizophrenic with greater frequency than men. This disorder, particularly associated with the drift phenomenon, seemingly has little relevance to women's social class as reflected by their neighborhood of residence.

c) Marital Status

The findings in this area are of interest mainly because they confirm previous findings. There appears to be little doubt that married persons utilize mental hospitals at a lower rate than persons who are not married. Never-married persons show a higher hospital utilization rate than persons who have been widowed, divorced, or separated. It would appear that marriage lowers one's risk of being hospitalized with a psychiatric disorder. This is interpreted to be mainly attributable to some protective qualities of the family. It is also possible that persons fail to marry and are admitted to mental hospitals for the same general reason, i.e., emotional disorder. This latter explanation is weakened by the elevated admission rates for the widowed, divorced, and separated persons who did in fact marry but have been reinstated in a high risk category by virtue of the dissolution of the family unit. The fantasticly elevated admission rate from the Loop (C.A. 32) for both first admissions and readmissions attests in part to the vulnerability of isolated and detached persons to mental hospitalization. The absence of family structure is one potent aspect of an extrusion bias.

d) Race

Race per se does not appear to be significantly involved in determining risk of mental hospitalization. Other factors, such as poverty or residence in a socially disorganized area, or an area undergoing rapid social change, are related both to increased risk of mental hospitalization and to race. That nonwhite rates of mental hospitalization are somewhat lower than white rates in proportion to representation in the population of Chicago appears to us to be related to a higher risk of arrest and imprisonment for blacks than for whites for equivalent behavior. A very interesting finding with regard to race is that black admissions appear to be highest in those areas which have the smallest percentage of black residents. It would appear that blacks living in predominantly white areas are at greater risk of mental hospitalization than blacks living in all-black areas. The same would hold for whites living in predominantly black areas. Blacks, regardless of sex, when admitted to a psychiatric facility typically receive a more severe diagnosis (schizophrenia). White males more often receive the diagnosis of alcoholism. White females more often receive the diagnoses of schizophrenia and psychophysiologic, psychoneurotic, and personality disorder.

e) Social Class

Prevalence of serious psychiatric disorder, in particular, schizophrenia, diseases of the senium, and alcoholism, is found to be associated with residents of communities which are poor and socially unstable. Poverty will determine whether one attends a public or private facility for treatment. It is hypothesized that the poor receive less adequate care for a first episode of emotional disorder, are more prone to acquire permanent disability, and either stay fixed at a low point in the social structure or sink lower. Psychoneurosis and manic-depressive psychosis tend to be associated with higher socio-economic class. Data from other sources tend to attribute this to the attitudes and habits of psychiatrists with regard to diagnosis and the social class of the patient. Our data tend to support this view and lead us to the conclusion that there is probably no true link between social class and the incidence of any psychiatric disorder.

f) Diagnosis

Of particular interest is the contrast between our findings with regard to diagnosis of first admissions with those of Faris and Dunham done in Chicago some thirty years earlier. The only area of obvious disagreement is the distribution of schizophrenic first admissions. Our results show schizophrenic first admissions to be distributed in random fashion over the city while Faris and Dunham found a definite concentration in the city center and moreover that the admission rates abated in all directions from the city center to the city perimeter. Later findings by Dunham (1965) based on research in Detroit on schizophrenia did not corroborate his Chicago findings and indeed facilitated an important shift in his thinking from a social causation to a social selection hypothesis as described in Chapter 1. The findings reported in *Community and Schizophrenia* (1965) are compatible with our findings with regard to schizophrenia. Still the patterning of unduplicated admissions does approximate very well Faris and Dunham's original finding for first admission schizophrenics. This is explained by our study tapping into a "latent" middle-class schizophrenic population because of our coverage of psychiatric units of general hospitals which were largely nonexistent at the time of the Faris and Dunham study. The juxtaposition of patterns between first admission and unduplicated admission (readmission) schizophrenics is our strongest bit of evidence in favor of a drift phenomenon in this disorder.

In other respects the two studies do agree. For total first admissions (all disorders), manic-depressive psycho-

sis, alcoholism, and diseases of the senium the distributions are similar. Total first admissions and unduplicated admissions show a concentration in the city center
and a tendency to abate as one moves to the outer perimeter. Manic-depressive first admissions and unduplicated admissions tend (weakly) to come from middle-
class areas and thus tend to show a fairly random pattern throughout the city. Alcoholism first admissions
and unduplicated admissions concentrate in the city center and tend to fall off as one proceeds to the periphery.
Senile first and unduplicated admissions cluster in the
city center but do not show any uniform decline away
from the city center. Hospitalization for this disorder is
strongly related to poverty. Additionally, psychophysiologic, psychoneurotic, and personality disorder first and
unduplicated admissions show a scattering throughout
the city. If any trend is discernible, it is a tendency for
such admissions to be correlated with middle-class social
credentials at the time of first admission. However, readmission patterns weaken this trend in that admissions
come from both lower- and middle-class communities.

g) Social Change

Much evidence is available to support the contention
that social change is correlated with mental hospital admission rates. The literature on migration and mental illness, while not unanimous on this point, does tend to
implicate relocation with an elevated risk for developing
a mental illness (See, for example, Murphy, 1961, and
Kantor, 1965). The breakdown of old communities due to
urban renewal (Fried, 1963) causes the suspension of established systems of social support; this could be expected to precipitate emotional disorder in persons who
might otherwise continue to function well. The risks of
rapid social change are particularly great for older per-

sons but are apparently quite general for all ages. In our study it is precisely those areas of the city which are undergoing rapid and drastic social change which appear to create the highest rates of psychiatric casualties.

h) Racial and Ethnic Composition of Communities

One manifestation of social change which is highly visible in large cities like Chicago is the change in the racial and ethnic composition of a neighborhood. Beyond this, minority status per se in a community area elevates the risk for mental hospital admission. Conversely, it is the all white areas where rates of unduplicated admission are lowest and the black areas where rates of first admission are lowest.

i) Poverty

The old villain poverty emerges in our study, once again, as a significant factor related to the prevalence of serious mental disorder. It would appear, however, that the relationship is not causal. Poverty does not relate in any clear fashion to incidence. The poor would appear to develop mental disorders with similar frequency as the well-off, but are less successfully treated and maintained in a functional status. As a side issue one might recall that on occasion the criterion of social competence is invoked as a measure of mental illness for the poor, but considered as an inadequate criterion for the well-off. One might consider that mental illness results in decreased social competence in the poor because of inadequate treatment while the ravages of mental illness are better contained in members of the middle class. The phenomenon, instrumentally related to the phenomenon of drift or social selection, causes an accumulation of cases (increased prevalence) of serious mental disorder in the lower classes and thus in lower-class neighborhoods.

j) Extrusion

Finally, the phenomenon of extrusion bias appears to be critical when one's measure of psychiatric casualties is mental hospital admissions. Communities vary in their propensity to push out or hold on to persons with given kinds and degrees of mental disorder. It may turn out that this property of communities is more significant in determining rates of mental hospital utilization (or other institutional use patterns) than any standard characterization of the properties of a patient ripe for mental hospitalization. It is interesting to reflect parenthetically on the standard criteria for admission to a mental hospital: "dangerous to self ... dangerous to others ... incapable of managing his own affairs ..." Such criteria, as our friends in the legal profession are bound to point out, are extremely vague and allow for a maximum of interpretation on the part of the person making the judgment. It could be argued that the criteria are vague for the same reason that such vague (and lately thought to be unconstitutional) laws against vagrancy and loitering are put on the books. Vagueness allows selective enforcement of the law at the discretion of the police. Similarly, vague criteria for mental hospitalization allow discretion on the part of communities as to who goes into a hospital and who is handled in the community by other means. Extrusion bias is a characteristic of a community which is determined by the cohesiveness of its social structure, the presence and intactness of interpersonal support systems, and its characteristic attitudes towards mental illness and psychiatry.

BIBLIOGRAPHY

Anderson, N. *The hobo*. Chicago: University of Chicago Press, Phoenix Books, 1961.

Bogue, D. J. *Skid row in American cities*. Chicago: Community and Family Study Center, 1963.

Burgess, E. W., and Bogue, D. J. (Eds.). *Contributions to urban sociology*. Chicago: University of Chicago Press, 1963.

Chicago, Welfare Council of, *Chicago community area profiles*. Chicago: Research Department, Welfare Council of Metropolitan Chicago, Publication No. 4006, 1964.

Clausen, J. A., and Kohn, M. L. The ecological approach in social psychiatry. *American Journal of Sociology,* 1954, 60, 140-151.

Clausen, J. A., and Kohn, M. L. Relation of schizophrenia to the social structure of a small city. In B. Pasamanick (Ed.), *Epidemiology of mental disorders*. Washington, D.C.: American Association for the Advancement of Science, Publication No. 60, 1959.

Dawson, W. R. Presidential address on the relation between the geographical distribution of insanity and that of certain social and other conditions in Ireland. *Journal of Mental Science,* 1911, 57, 571-597.

Deas, P. M. An illustration of local differences in the distribution of insanity. *Journal of Mental Science,* 1875, 21, 61-67.

Dohrenwend, B. P., and Dohrenwend, B. S. *Social status and psychological disorder: A causal inquiry*. New York: Wiley-Interscience, 1969.

Dunham, H. W. *Sociological theory and mental disorders*. Detroit: Wayne State University Press, 1959.

Dunham, H. W. Social structures and mental disorders: competing hypotheses of explanation. In *Causes of mental disor-*

ders: a review of epidemiological knowledge. New York: Milbank Memorial Fund, 1961.

Dunham, H. W. *Community and schizophrenia.* Detroit: Wayne State University Press, 1965.

Dunham, H. W. Epidemiology of psychiatric disorders as a contribution to medical ecology. *Archives of General Psychiatry,* 1966, 14, 1-19.

Faris, R. E. L., and Dunham, H. W. *Mental disorders in urban areas.* New York: Hafner Publishing Co., 1960.

Festinger, L. Laboratory experiments. In L. Festinger and D. Katz (Eds.), *Research methods in the behavioral sciences.* New York: Dryden Press, 1953.

Fried, M. Grieving for a lost home. In L. Duhl (Ed.), *The urban condition.* New York: Basic Books, 1963.

Gerard, D. L., and Houston, L. G. Family setting and the social ecology of schizophrenia. *Psychiatric Quarterly,* 1953, 27, 90-101.

Grunfeld, B., and Salversen, C. Functional psychoses and social status. *British Journal of Psychiatry,* 1968, 114, 733-737.

Hafner, H., and Reimann, H. Spatial distribution of mental disorders in Mannheim, 1965. In E. H. Hare and J. K. Wing (Eds.), *Psychiatric epidemiology.* London: Oxford Press, 1970.

Hollingshead, A. B., and Redlich, F. C. Schizophrenia and social structure. *American Journal of Psychiatry,* 1954, 110, 695-701.

Hollingshead, A. B., and Redlich, F. C. *Social class and mental illness.* New York: Wiley and Sons, Science Editions, 1958.

Hughes, C., Tremblay, M., Rapoport, R., and Leighton, A. *People of cove and woodlot.* New York: Basic Books, 1960.

Juel-Nielsen, N., and Stromgren, E. *Five years later: A comparison between census studies of patients in psychiatric institutions in Denmark in 1957 and 1962.* Copenhagen: Munksgaard, 1963.

Kantor, M. B. (Ed.). *Mobility and mental health.* Springfield, Ill.: Thomas, 1965.

Kitagawa, E. M., and Taeuber, K. E. (Eds.). *Local community fact book: Chicago metropolitan area, 1960.* Chicago: University of Chicago, 1963.

Kramer, M. Some problems for international research suggested by observations on differences in first admission rates to mental hospitals in England and Wales and of the United States. Montreal: Proceedings of the Third World Congress of Psychiatry, 1961, p. 153.

Langner, T. S., and Michael, S. T. *Life stress and mental health.* New York: Free Press of Glencoe, 1963.

LaPouse, R., Monk, M., and Terris, M. The drift hypothesis and socioeconomic differentials in schizophrenia. *American Journal of Public Health,* 1956, 46, 978-986.

Leighton, A. H. *My name is legion.* New York: Basic Books, 1959.

Leighton, D., Harding, J., Macklin, D., Macmillan, A., and Leighton, A. *The character of danger: Psychiatric symptoms in selected communities.* New York: Basic Books, 1963.

Levy, L. An evaluation of the Illinois mental health program, 1960-1970, by the use of selected operating statistics. *American Journal of Public Health,* 1971, 61, 2038-2045.

Lin, T. The epidemiological study of mental disorders by WHO. *Social Psychiatry,* 1967, 1, 204.

MacDermott, W. R. The topographical distribution of insanity. *British Medical Journal,* 1908, 2, 950.

Maris, R. *Social forces in urban suicide.* Homewood, Ill.: Dorsey Press, 1969.

Menzel, H. Comments on Robinson's "Ecological correlations and the behavior of individuals." In S. M. Lipset and N. J. Smelser (Eds.), *Sociology: The progress of a decade.* Englewood Cliffs, New Jersey: Prentice-Hall, 1961.

Murphy, H. M. B. Social change and mental health. *Milbank Memorial Fund Quarterly,* 1961, 39, 385-445.

Myerson, A. Review of "Mental disorders in Urban areas." *American Journal of Psychiatry,* 1940, 96, 995-997.

Park, R. E. The city. *Human communities.* Glencoe, Ill.: The Free Press, 1952.

Pugh, T., and MacMahon, B. *Epidemiologic findings in United States mental hospital data.* Boston: Little, Brown and Co., 1962.

Queen, S. A. The ecological study of mental disorders. *American Sociological Review,* 1940, 5, 201-209.

Robinson, W. S. Ecological correlations and the behavior of individuals. In S. M. Lipset and N. J. Smelser (Eds.), *Sociology: The progress of a decade.* Englewood Cliffs, New Jersey, Prentice-Hall, 1961.

Schroeder, C. W. Mental disorders in cities. *American Journal of Sociology,* 1942, 48, 40-47.

Srole, L., Langner, T. S., Michael, S. T., Opler, M. K., and Rennie, T. A. C. *Mental health in the metropolis: The midtown Manhattan study.* New York: McGraw-Hill, 1962.

Stein, L. Social class gradient in schizophrenia. *British Journal of Preventive and Social Medicine,* 1957, 2, 181-195.

Stein, M. R. *The Eclipse of Community.* Evanston: Harper and Row, 1964.

Stengel, E. Classification of mental diseases. *Bulletin of the World Health Organization,* 1960, 21, 601.

Sutherland, J. F. *The growth and geographical distribution of lunacy in Scotland.* Glasgow: British Association for the Advancement of Science, Sept. 1901.

Thrasher, F. *The gang.* Chicago: University of Chicago Press, 1927.

Turner, R., and Wagenfeld, M. Occupational mobility and schizophrenia: An assessment of the social causation and social selection hypotheses. *American Sociological Review,* 1967, 32, 104-113.

United States Dept. of Health, Education, and Welfare. *Characteristics of patients in mental hospitals, United States—April-June, 1963.* Washington, D.C.: 1965.

White, W. The geographical distribution of insanity in the United States. *Journal of Nervous and Mental Disorders,* 1903, 30, 257-279.

Wirth, L. *The ghetto.* Chicago: University of Chicago Press, 1928.

Wirth, L., and Furez, M. (Eds.). *Local community fact book, 1938.* Chicago: Chicago Recreation Commission, 1938.

Wright, A. The increase of insanity. *Conference on Charities and Corrections,* 1884, 228-236.

Zorbaugh, H. *The gold coast and the slum.* Chicago: University of Chicago Press, 1929.

Appendix A

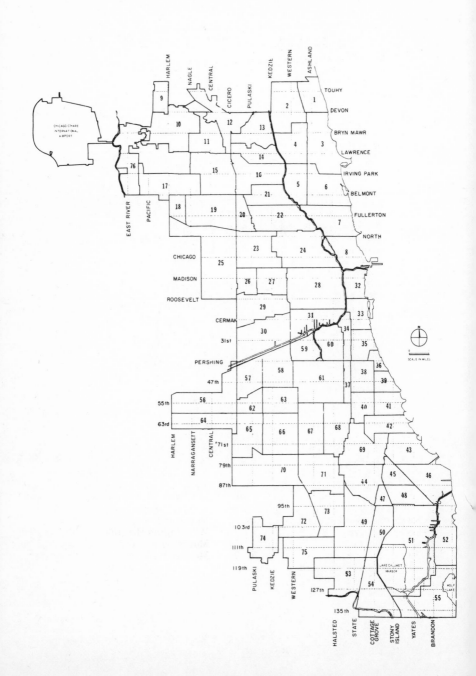

COMMUNITY AREAS
CITY OF CHICAGO
1960

No.	Name	No.	Name
1	Rogers Park	39	Kenwood
2	West Ridge	40	Washington Park
3	Uptown	41	Hyde Park
4	Lincoln Square	42	Woodlawn
5	North Center	43	South Shore
6	Lakeview	44	Chatham
7	Lincoln Park	45	Avalon Park
8	Near North Side	46	South Chicago
9	Edison Park	47	Burnside
10	Norwood Park	48	Calumet Heights
11	Jefferson Park	49	Roseland
12	Forest Glen	50	Pullman
13	North Park	51	South Deering
14	Albany Park	52	East Side
15	Portage Park	53	West Pullman
16	Irving Park	54	Riverdale
17	Dunning	55	Hegewisch
18	Montclare	56	Garfield Ridge
19	Belmont Cragin	57	Archer Heights
20	Hermosa	58	Brighton Park
21	Avondale	59	McKinley Park
22	Logan Square	60	Bridgeport
23	Humboldt Park	61	New City
24	West Town	62	West Elsdon
25	Austin	63	Gage Park
26	West Garfield Park	64	Clearing
27	East Garfield Park	65	West Lawn
28	Near West Side	66	Chicago Lawn
29	North Lawndale	67	West Englewood
30	South Lawndale	68	Englewood
31	Lower West Side	69	Greater Grand Crossing
32	Loop	70	Ashburn
33	Near South Side	71	Auburn Gresham
34	Armour Square	72	Beverly
35	Douglas	73	Washington Heights
36	Oakland	74	Mount Greenwood
37	Fuller Park	75	Morgan Park
38	Grand Boulevard		

Appendix B

TABLE B-1
Unduplicated Admission Rates
per 100,000 Adult Population, by Sex

C.A.	Males Number Admitted	Male Pop.	Rate	Females Number Admitted	Female Pop.	Rate
City Totals	5,283	1,240,445	425.8	5129	1,344,713	381.4
1	74	20584	359.5	140	26010	538.3
2	54	23246	232.3	113	26384	428.3
3	255	49382	516.4	320	55674	574.8
4	70	18011	388.7	73	21899	333.4
5	40	15579	256.8	52	17881	290.8
6	152	44325	342.9	229	51284	446.5
7	149	33122	449.9	161	34693	464.1
8	258	29015	889.2	194	28516	680.3
9	7	4162	168.2	17	4726	359.7
10	24	14246	168.5	31	15840	195.7
11	13	10068	129.1	35	11038	317.1
12	15	6909	217.1	17	7774	218.7
13	20	6656	300.5	32	7429	430.7
14	46	18106	254.1	109	20262	538.0
15	61	23985	254.3	88	27180	323.8
16	53	21175	250.3	79	23927	330.2
17	31	14985	206.9	56	16223	345.2
18	7	4346	161.1	17	4807	353.7
19	60	22583	265.7	84	24770	339.1
20	19	7792	243.8	34	8655	392.8
21	38	14285	266.0	42	15724	267.1
22	129	34111	378.2	131	35666	367.3
23	78	25656	304.0	104	27236	381.9
24	212	50016	423.9	188	48250	389.6
25	148	45010	328.8	209	52734	396.3
26	68	15542	437.5	54	16085	335.7
27	98	20652	474.5	74	21173	349.5
28	722	43852	1646.5	154	36447	422.5
29	109	33721	323.2	104	38679	268.9
30	74	23101	320.3	86	22499	382.2
31	58	17062	339.9	62	16471	376.4
32	219	3581	6115.6	20	699	2861.2
33	32	3241	987.3	16	3019	530.0
34	25	5128	487.5	17	5046	336.9
35	81	14890	544.0	72	17296	416.3
36	31	6293	492.6	29	7703	376.5
37	9	3463	259.9	14	3842	364.4
38	139	27197	511.1	90	30754	292.6

TABLE B-1 (Continued)
Unduplicated Admission Rates
per 100,000 Adult Population, by Sex

C.A.	Males Number Admitted	Male Pop.	Rate	Females Number Admitted	Female Pop.	Rate
39	44	13449	327.2	61	15272	399.4
40	83	16008	518.5	60	17744	338.1
41	93	17166	541.8	98	18884	519.0
42	127	27669	459.0	134	30035	446.2
43	103	26565	387.7	160	33388	479.2
44	51	15065	338.5	52	17231	301.8
45	12	4451	269.6	18	4933	364.9
46	54	17819	303.1	56	18293	306.1
47	6	1256	477.7	3	1233	243.3
48	14	6648	210.6	20	6941	288.1
49	48	20561	233.5	72	22590	318.7
50	16	3084	518.8	9	3050	295.1
51	21	6183	339.6	28	6164	454.3
52	17	8474	200.6	19	8314	228.5
53	22	12110	181.7	21	12689	165.5
54	10	2091	478.2	9	2850	315.8
55	5	3211	155.7	8	3033	263.8
56	15	12868	116.6	59	13405	440.1
57	7	3822	183.1	15	3989	376.0
58	38	13955	272.3	36	14294	251.9
59	17	5936	286.4	14	6199	225.8
60	68	14322	474.8	56	14789	378.7
61	121	23276	519.9	97	24000	404.2
62	17	4956	343.0	15	5508	272.3
63	34	10519	323.2	35	11479	304.9
64	15	6433	233.2	13	6368	204.2
65	13	9402	138.3	30	10035	299.0
66	56	19369	289.1	62	21603	287.0
67	88	20330	432.9	85	22271	381.7
68	149	30081	495.3	113	33271	339.6
69	54	21268	253.9	70	24042	291.2
70	14	11333	123.5	30	12022	249.5
71	77	21362	360.5	82	25173	325.8
72	19	8249	230.3	45	9775	460.4
73	36	10195	353.1	41	11618	352.9
74	15	6856	218.8	24	7577	316.8
75	26	9025	288.1	32	10356	309.0

TABLE B-2
Black and White Hospital Utilization Rates
per 100,000 Adult Population

C.A.	White Pop.	No. White	Rate	Black Pop.	No. Black	Rate
City Totals	2,712,748	3,486	312.8	812,637	1,909	234.9
1	56,503	212	375.2	57	1	1754.4
2	63,696	167	262.2	81	0	0.0
3	122,595	564	460.1	423	8	1891.3
4	49,544	142	286.6	30	0	0.0
5	43,622	92	210.9	48	0	0.0
6	115,018	379	329.5	168	1	595.2
7	84,604	303	358.1	1,358	6	441.8
8	50,569	388	767.3	23,114	62	268.2
9	12,565	24	191.0	0	0	0.0
10	40,915	55	134.4	12	0	0.0
11	27,475	48	174.3	0	0	0.0
12	19,203	32	166.6	6	0	0.0
13	17,280	52	300.9	517	0	0.0
14	49,250	155	314.7	19	0	0.0
15	65,841	148	224.8	17	1	5882.4
16	58,125	129	221.9	20	3	1500.0
17	41,560	87	209.3	2	0	0.0
18	11,785	24	203.7	1	0	0.0
19	60,838	144	236.7	3	0	0.0
20	21,401	53	247.7	0	0	0.0
21	39,613	80	202.0	3	0	0.0
22	94,076	260	276.4	371	0	0.0
23	70,972	181	255.0	425	1	235.3
24	136,479	392	287.2	2,366	8	338.1
25	124,916	357	285.8	31	0	0.0
26	38,152	107	280.5	7,204	15	208.2
27	25,409	74	291.2	41,097	97	236.0
28	57,676	696	1206.7	68,146	179	262.7
29	10,792	40	370.7	113,827	173	152.0
30	57,278	155	270.6	3,568	5	140.1
31	47,795	117	244.8	530	2	377.4
32	3,841	227	5909.9	449	12	2672.6
33	2,354	20	849.6	7,942	28	352.6
34	9,096	26	285.8	4,960	14	282.3
35	3,880	17	438.1	48,031	136	283.2
36	311	4	1286.2	23,955	56	233.8
37	476	3	630.3	11,692	20	171.1
38	398	13	3266.3	79,537	216	271.6
39	6,282	27	429.8	34,838	77	221.0
40	332	13	3915.7	43,310	130	300.2

TABLE B-2 (Continued)
Black and White Hospital Utilization Rates
per 100,000 Adult Population

C.A.	White Pop.	No. White	Rate	Black Pop.	No. Black	Rate
41	27,214	156	573.2	17,163	35	203.9
42	8,450	58	686.4	72,397	203	280.4
43	65,507	249	380.1	7,018	14	199.5
44	15,090	37	245.2	26,756	66	246.7
45	12,660	30	237.0	6	0	0.0
46	47,338	107	226.0	2,448	3	122.5
47	3,454	9	260.6	0	0	0.0
48	19,313	32	165.7	8	2	25000.0
49	45,392	100	220.3	13,255	20	150.9
50	8,400	25	297.6	0	0	0.0
51	18,637	47	252.2	125	2	1600.0
52	23,191	36	155.2	4	0	0.0
53	35,328	43	121.7	62	0	0.0
54	1,127	1	88.7	10,306	18	174.7
55	8,900	13	146.1	32	0	0.0
56	37,675	73	193.8	2,686	1	37.2
57	10,583	22	207.9	1	0	0.0
58	37,948	74	195.0	36	0	0.0
59	16,885	31	183.6	0	0	0.0
60	41,436	121	292.0	65	2	3076.9
61	67,172	215	320.1	1666	2	1204.8
62	14,210	32	225.2	0	0	0.0
63	28,222	69	244.5	2	0	0.0
64	18,777	28	149.1	2	0	0.0
65	26,893	43	159.9	5	0	0.0
66	51,294	118	230.0	3	0	0.0
67	51,583	155	300.5	6,842	18	263.1
68	30,107	120	398.6	67,216	142	211.3
69	8,687	24	276.3	54,257	100	184.3
70	38,604	44	114.0	1	0	0.0
71	59,346	159	267.9	91	0	0.0
72	24,791	63	254.1	14	1	7142.9
73	26,017	65	249.8	3,711	12	323.4
74	21,918	39	149.9	4	0	0.0
75	18,082	41	226.7	9,797	17	173.5

TABLE B-3
Age Distributions and Unduplicated Admissions by Age for the 75 Chicago Community Areas

	Age Distribution of Community Area Populations										Admission Populations by Age										
	C.A. Pop.	% (To-tal)	0-24	%	25-44	%	45-64	%	65+	%	Un-dup. Ad-miss.	% (To-tal)	0-24	%	25-44	%	45-64	%	65+	%
1	56,888	100	17,629	30.9	14,377	25.3	16,830	29.6	8,052	14.2	214	100	18	8.4	60	28.0	92	43.0	44	20.6
2	63,884	100	22,338	35.0	15,084	23.5	19,893	31.2	6,569	10.3	167	100	27	16.2	53	31.7	57	34.1	30	18.0
3	127,682	100	38,148	29.9	33,613	26.3	37,040	29.0	18,881	14.8	575	100	32	5.5	200	34.8	216	37.6	127	22.1
4	49,850	100	15,862	31.8	12,225	24.5	15,088	30.3	6,675	13.4	143	100	10	6.9	46	32.2	63	44.1	24	16.8
5	43,877	100	15,861	36.2	10,950	25.0	11,565	26.4	5,501	12.4	92	100	6	6.5	32	34.8	39	42.4	15	16.3
6	118,764	100	37,484	31.6	31,354	26.4	34,558	29.1	15,368	12.9	381	100	26	6.8	127	33.3	166	43.6	62	16.3
7	88,836	100	32,936	37.1	24,819	27.9	21,214	23.9	9,867	11.1	320	100	22	7.1	126	40.7	116	37.4	46	14.8
8	75,509	100	28,106	37.2	21,109	28.0	18,606	24.6	7,688	10.2	452	100	31	6.8	191	42.3	176	38.9	54	12.0
9	12,568	100	4,891	39.0	3,109	24.7	3,343	26.6	1,225	9.7	24	100	2	8.3	6	25.0	10	41.7	6	25.0
10	40,953	100	15,514	37.9	10,398	25.4	11,356	27.7	3,685	9.0	55	100	6	10.9	16	29.1	21	38.2	12	21.8
11	27,494	100	9,545	34.7	7,097	25.8	7,740	28.2	3,112	11.3	48	100	1	2.0	20	41.7	18	37.5	9	18.8
12	19,228	100	6,632	34.5	4,138	21.5	6,618	34.4	1,840	9.6	32	100	5	15.6	10	31.3	10	31.3	7	21.8
13	17,866	100	6,380	35.7	4,028	22.5	5,558	31.2	1,900	10.6	52	100	4	7.7	16	30.8	26	50.0	6	11.5
14	49,450	100	17,053	34.5	11,458	23.1	13,782	27.9	7,157	14.5	155	100	15	9.7	45	29.0	63	40.7	32	20.6
15	65,925	100	22,422	34.0	16,200	24.6	18,655	28.3	8,648	13.1	149	100	13	8.7	55	36.9	54	36.2	27	18.2
16	58,298	100	20,606	35.4	14,620	25.1	15,932	27.3	7,140	12.2	132	100	12	9.1	43	32.6	54	40.9	23	17.4
17	41,626	100	15,605	37.5	10,591	25.4	11,640	28.0	3,790	9.1	87	100	9	10.4	32	36.8	31	35.6	15	17.2
18	11,802	100	4,151	35.2	2,908	24.6	3,310	28.0	1,433	12.2	24	100	2	8.3	10	41.7	10	41.7	2	8.3
19	60,883	100	21,017	34.5	16,044	26.4	16,468	27.0	7,354	12.1	144	100	6	4.1	60	41.7	54	37.5	24	16.7
20	21,429	100	7,633	35.6	5,542	25.8	5,713	26.7	2,541	11.9	53	100	2	3.8	15	28.3	23	43.4	13	24.5
21	39,748	100	14,655	36.9	10,839	27.2	9,885	24.9	4,369	11.0	80	100	8	10.0	29	36.2	35	43.8	8	10.0
22	94,799	100	36,465	38.5	26,018	27.4	22,287	23.5	10,029	10.6	260	100	24	9.2	90	34.6	105	40.4	41	15.8
23	71,609	100	27,907	39.0	20,070	28.0	16,519	23.1	7,113	9.9	182	100	13	7.1	67	36.8	72	39.6	30	16.5

TABLE B-3 (Continued)
Age Distributions and Unduplicated Admissions by Age for the 75 Chicago Community Areas

	Age Distribution of Community Area Populations										Admission Populations by Age									
C.A.	Pop.	% (To-tal)	0-24	%	25-44	%	45-64	%	65+	%	Un-dup. Ad-miss.	% (To-tal)	0-24	%	25-44	%	45-64	%	65+	%
24	139,657	100	59,547	42.6	40,020	28.7	27,740	19.9	12,350	8.8	400	100	27	6.8	186	46.4	142	35.5	45	11.3
25	125,133	100	42,613	34.1	30,791	24.5	35,362	28.3	16,367	13.1	357	100	17	4.8	108	30.3	155	43.3	77	21.6
26	45,611	100	20,934	45.9	12,541	27.5	8,449	18.5	3,687	8.1	122	100	10	8.1	54	44.3	39	32.0	19	15.6
27	66,871	100	35,472	53.0	19,751	29.6	8,646	12.9	3,002	4.5	172	100	35	20.3	72	41.9	44	25.6	21	12.2
28	126,610	100	63,436	50.1	34,799	27.5	21,057	16.6	7,318	5.8	876	100	40	4.6	362	41.3	381	43.5	93	10.6
29	124,937	100	70,636	56.5	35,301	28.3	14,860	11.9	4,140	3.3	213	100	33	15.5	111	52.1	48	22.5	21	9.9
30	60,940	100	23,277	38.2	17,075	28.0	14,339	23.5	6,249	10.3	160	100	14	8.8	65	40.5	62	38.8	19	11.9
31	48,448	100	21,216	43.8	13,723	28.3	9,191	19.0	4,318	8.9	120	100	6	5.0	58	48.3	36	30.0	20	16.7
32	4,337	100	442	10.2	1,268	29.2	1,766	40.7	861	19.9	239	100	7	2.9	81	33.9	132	55.2	19	8.0
33	10,350	100	5,324	51.4	2,659	25.7	1,532	14.8	835	8.1	48	100	6	12.5	21	43.8	17	35.4	4	8.3
34	15,783	100	7,640	48.4	4,188	26.5	2,649	16.8	1,306	8.3	42	100	8	19.1	17	40.4	12	28.6	5	11.9
35	52,325	100	26,735	51.0	14,105	27.0	8,294	15.9	3,191	6.1	153	100	22	14.4	84	54.9	28	18.3	19	12.4
36	24,378	100	13,306	54.6	6,408	26.3	3,512	14.4	1,152	4.7	60	100	5	8.4	30	50.0	17	28.3	8	13.3
37	12,181	100	6,457	53.0	3,179	26.1	2,015	16.5	530	4.4	23	100	5	21.7	10	43.5	6	26.1	2	8.7
38	80,036	100	30,916	38.6	21,611	27.0	20,018	25.0	7,491	9.4	228	100	21	9.2	104	45.6	64	28.1	39	17.1
39	41,533	100	18,241	43.9	13,352	32.2	7,477	18.0	2,463	5.9	105	100	14	13.3	53	50.5	23	21.9	15	14.3
40	43,690	100	14,694	33.6	12,728	29.1	12,042	27.6	4,226	9.7	143	100	17	11.8	67	46.9	38	26.6	21	14.7
41	45,577	100	16,489	36.2	13,886	30.4	9,931	21.8	5,271	11.6	191	100	26	13.6	81	42.4	56	29.3	28	14.7
42	81,279	100	34,402	42.4	26,770	32.9	14,989	18.4	5,118	6.3	261	100	30	11.5	124	47.5	70	26.8	37	14.2
43	73,086	100	20,880	28.6	16,327	22.3	24,374	33.4	11,505	15.7	263	100	24	9.1	76	28.9	127	48.3	36	13.7
44	41,962	100	14,716	35.1	13,199	31.5	10,376	24.7	3,671	8.7	103	100	12	11.7	57	55.2	22	21.4	12	11.7
45	12,710	100	4,767	37.5	2,990	23.5	3,523	27.7	1,430	11.3	30	100	2	6.7	11	36.6	12	40.0	5	16.7
46	49,913	100	20,134	40.3	12,961	26.0	12,119	24.3	4,699	9.4	110	100	9	8.2	32	29.1	52	47.2	17	15.5
47	3,463	100	1,399	40.3	975	28.2	744	21.5	345	10.0	9	.00	0	0.0	4	44.4	3	33.3	2	22.3

171

TABLE B-3 (Continued)

Age Distributions and Unduplicated Admissions by Age for the 75 Chicago Community Areas

| | Age Distribution of Community Area Populations | | | | | | | | | | Admission Populations by Age | | | | | | | | | | |
| | | % (To-tal) | 0-24 | % | 25-44 | % | 45-64 | % | 65+ | % | Un-dup. Ad-miss. (To-tal) | % (To-tal) | 0-24 | % | 25-44 | % | 45-64 | % | 65+ | % |
C.A.	Pop.																			
48	19,352	100	7,786	40.2	5,733	29.6	4,432	22.9	1,401	7.3	34	100	2	5.9	14	41.2	13	38.2	5	14.7
49	58,750	100	22,650	38.6	14,344	24.4	15,506	26.4	6,250	10.6	120	100	11	9.2	40	33.3	50	41.7	19	15.8
50	8,412	100	3,275	38.9	2,271	27.1	2,105	25.0	761	9.0	25	100	3	12.0	9	36.0	10	40.0	3	12.0
51	18,794	100	8,575	45.6	5,601	29.8	3,437	18.3	1,181	6.3	49	100	4	10.2	21	42.9	17	34.7	6	12.2
52	23,214	100	9,451	40.7	6,286	27.1	5,615	24.2	1,862	8.0	36	100	2	5.6	12	33.3	16	44.4	6	16.7
53	35,397	100	14,710	41.5	9,821	27.8	7,728	21.8	3,138	8.9	43	100	6	14.0	17	39.4	14	32.6	6	14.0
54	11,448	100	7,946	69.4	2,418	21.1	777	6.8	307	2.7	19	100	7	36.8	9	47.4	2	10.5	1	5.3
55	8,936	100	3,862	43.2	2,672	29.9	1,728	19.3	674	7.6	13	100	2	15.4	6	46.1	5	38.5	0	0.0
56	40,449	100	18,713	46.3	12,969	32.1	6,848	16.9	1,919	4.7	74	100	2	2.7	29	39.2	27	36.5	16	21.6
57	10,584	100	4,019	38.0	3,254	30.7	2,206	20.8	1,105	10.5	22	100	4	18.2	11	50.0	4	13.6	4	18.2
58	38,019	100	14,771	38.9	10,995	28.9	8,326	21.9	3,927	10.3	74	100	5	6.8	32	43.2	27	36.5	10	13.5
59	16,908	100	6,984	41.3	4,668	27.6	3,654	21.6	1,602	9.5	31	100	7	22.5	11	35.5	11	35.5	2	6.5
60	41,560	100	17,912	43.1	11,332	27.3	8,396	20.2	3,920	9.4	124	100	8	6.5	61	49.1	45	36.3	10	8.1
61	67,428	100	29,555	43.8	18,647	27.7	13,291	19.7	5,935	8.8	218	100	19	8.7	92	42.2	81	37.2	26	11.9
62	14,215	100	5,543	40.0	4,240	28.8	3,415	24.0	1,017	7.2	32	100	3	9.4	13	40.6	13	40.6	3	9.4
63	28,244	100	9,899	35.1	7,274	25.7	7,681	27.2	3,390	12.0	69	100	9	13.1	21	30.4	22	31.9	17	24.6
64	18,797	100	8,544	45.4	6,010	32.0	3,346	17.8	897	4.8	28	100	3	10.7	15	53.6	9	32.1	1	3.6
65	26,910	100	10,662	39.6	7,972	29.6	6,265	23.3	2,011	7.5	43	100	2	4.6	18	41.9	20	46.5	3	7.0
66	51,347	100	16,694	32.5	12,565	24.5	15,755	30.7	6,333	12.3	118	100	10	8.4	46	39.0	37	31.4	25	21.2
67	58,516	100	23,827	40.7	14,765	25.2	13,630	23.3	6,294	10.8	173	100	15	8.7	67	38.7	55	31.8	36	20.8
68	97,595	100	47,797	49.0	26,500	27.1	16,779	17.2	6,519	6.7	263	100	22	8.7	130	49.3	80	30.3	31	11.7
69	63,169	100	25,485	40.4	19,385	30.7	13,865	21.9	4,434	7.0	124	100	17	13.7	58	46.8	32	25.8	17	13.7
70	38,638	100	18,402	47.6	12,742	33.0	5,988	15.5	1,506	3.9	44	100	2	4.6	23	52.2	16	36.4	3	6.8
71	59,484	100	20,107	33.8	12,852	21.7	18,162	30.4	8,363	14.1	159	100	9	5.6	40	25.2	70	44.0	40	25.2
72	24,814	100	9,366	37.7	4,809	19.4	7,673	30.9	2,966	12.0	64	100	3	4.7	19	29.7	30	46.9	12	18.7
73	29,793	100	11,264	37.8	7,180	24.1	8,155	27.4	3,194	10.7	77	100	5	6.5	23	29.9	35	45.4	14	18.2
74	21,941	100	10,189	46.4	5,989	27.3	4,517	20.6	1,246	5.7	39	100	3	7.7	14	35.9	14	35.9	8	20.5
75	27,912	100	11,776	42.2	6,428	23.0	6,747	24.2	2,961	10.6	58	100	1	1.7	27	46.6	23	39.6	7	12.1

TABLE B-4
Percentage Distribution of People Admitted to Public and Private Mental Hospitals by Community Area and Marital Status

C.A.	Totl.	Sgle.	%	Mar.	%	Wid.	%	Div.	%	Sep.	%	Unkn.	%
City Totals	10653	2957	27.8	3945	37.0	1196	11.2	1354	13.0	1068	10.0	133	1.2
1	214	54	25.2	97	45.3	31	14.5	19	8.9	11	5.1	2	0.9
2	167	40	24.0	89	53.3	24	14.4	8	4.8	4	2.4	2	1.2
3	575	143	25.0	204	35.5	78	13.6	94	16.3	45	7.8	11	1.9
4	143	41	29.0	69	48.3	15	10.5	13	9.1	5	3.5	0	0.0
5	92	20	21.7	45	48.9	7	7.6	14	15.2	5	5.4	1	1.1
6	381	104	27.3	160	42.0	41	10.8	46	12.1	29	7.6	1	0.3
7	310	98	32.6	95	30.6	42	13.5	49	15.8	22	7.1	4	1.3
8	452	136	30.1	106	23.5	39	8.6	95	21.0	69	15.3	7	1.5
9	24	6	25.0	12	50.0	5	20.8	0	0.0	0	0.0	1	4.2
10	55	16	29.1	30	54.5	6	10.9	1	1.8	2	3.6	0	0.0
11	48	7	15.0	31	64.6	9	18.8	1	2.1	0	0.0	0	0.0
12	32	10	31.3	11	34.4	8	25.0	3	9.4	0	0.0	0	0.0
13	52	11	21.2	27	51.9	6	11.5	3	5.8	5	9.6	0	0.0
14	155	35	22.6	81	52.3	24	15.5	10	6.5	5	3.2	0	0.0
15	149	48	32.2	72	48.3	14	9.4	8	5.4	4	2.7	3	2.0
16	132	30	22.7	60	45.5	19	14.4	15	11.4	8	6.1	0	0.0
17	87	17	19.5	50	57.5	9	10.3	7	8.0	4	4.6	0	0.0
18	24	5	20.8	13	54.2	3	12.5	2	8.3	0	0.0	1	4.2
19	144	29	20.1	84	58.3	18	12.5	7	4.9	5	3.5	1	0.7
20	53	9	17.0	32	60.4	6	11.3	3	5.7	3	5.7	0	0.0
21	80	21	26.3	45	56.3	8	10.0	4	5.0	2	2.5	0	0.0

TABLE B-4 (Continued)
Percentage Distribution of People Admitted to Public and Private Mental Hospitals by Community Area and Marital Status

C.A.	Totl.	Sgle.	%	Mar.	%	Wid.	%	Div.	%	Sep.	%	Unkn.	%
22	260	76	29.2	112	43.1	23	2.8	28	10.8	18	6.9	3	1.2
23	182	50	27.5	82	45.1	31	17.0	11	6.0	6	3.3	2	1.1
24	400	115	28.8	160	40.0	40	10.0	42	10.5	35	8.8	8	2.0
25	357	81	22.7	167	46.8	50	14.0	43	12.0	14	3.9	2	0.6
26	122	32	26.2	56	45.9	7	5.7	16	13.1	11	9.0	0	0.0
27	172	64	37.2	45	26.2	20	11.6	13	7.6	24	14.0	6	3.5
28	876	292	33.3	101	11.5	68	7.8	249	28.4	150	17.1	16	1.8
29	213	66	31.0	66	31.0	19	8.9	14	6.6	47	22.1	1	0.5
30	160	41	25.6	82	51.3	16	10.0	7	4.4	14	8.8	0	0.0
31	120	34	28.3	48	40.0	15	12.5	11	9.2	9	7.5	3	2.5
32	239	90	37.7	12	5.0	23	9.6	73	30.5	36	15.1	5	2.1
33	48	11	22.9	9	18.8	6	12.5	12	25.0	9	18.8	1	2.1
34	42	16	38.1	15	35.7	2	4.8	0	0.0	5	11.9	4	9.5
35	153	44	28.8	49	32.0	18	11.8	10	6.5	30	19.6	2	1.3
36	60	11	18.3	12	20.0	8	13.3	10	16.7	18	30.0	1	1.7
37	23	5	21.7	8	34.8	4	17.4	3	13.0	2	8.7	1	4.3
38	229	71	31.0	42	18.3	43	18.8	26	11.4	42	18.3	5	2.2
39	105	28	26.7	32	30.5	14	13.3	8	7.6	21	20.0	2	1.9
40	143	47	32.9	28	19.6	19	13.3	18	12.6	30	21.0	1	0.7
41	191	64	33.5	64	33.5	25	13.1	23	12.0	15	7.9	0	0.0
42	261	71	27.2	64	24.5	29	11.1	32	12.3	57	21.8	8	3.1
43	263	71	27.0	119	45.2	33	12.5	25	9.5	13	4.9	2	0.8
44	103	28	27.2	46	44.7	4	3.9	11	10.7	14	13.6	0	0.0
45	30	11	36.7	10	33.3	6	20.0	3	10.0	0	0.0	0	0.0

TABLE B-4 (Continued)
Percentage Distribution of People Admitted to Public and Private Mental Hospitals by Community Area and Marital Status

C.A.	Totl.	Sgle.	%	Mar.	%	Wid.	%	Div.	%	Sep.	%	Unkn.	%
46	110	32	29.1	49	44.5	11	10.0	8	7.3	10	9.1	0	0.0
47	9	2	22.2	3	33.3	2	22.2	2	22.2	0	0.0	0	0.0
48	34	6	17.6	24	70.6	1	2.9	1	2.9	1	2.9	1	2.9
49	120	25	20.8	62	51.7	12	10.0	12	10.0	8	6.7	1	0.8
50	25	8	32.0	10	40.0	1	4.0	5	20.0	1	4.0	0	0.0
51	49	11	22.4	30	61.2	4	8.2	2	4.1	2	4.1	0	0.0
52	36	10	27.8	21	58.3	2	5.6	2	5.6	0	0.0	1	2.8
52	43	4	9.3	28	65.1	2	4.7	5	11.6	2	4.7	2	4.7
54	19	6	31.6	7	36.8	0	0.0	1	5.3	5	26.3	0	0.0
55	13	4	30.8	7	53.8	1	7.7	0	0.0	1	7.7	0	0.0
56	74	14	18.9	38	51.4	14	18.9	6	8.1	2	2.7	0	0.0
57	22	7	31.8	12	54.5	3	13.6	0	0.0	0	0.0	0	0.0
58	74	23	31.1	34	45.9	4	5.4	4	5.4	7	9.5	2	2.7
59	31	12	38.7	17	54.8	0	0.0	2	6.5	0	0.0	0	0.0
60	124	38	30.6	57	46.0	10	8.1	11	8.9	7	5.6	1	0.8
61	218	62	28.4	84	38.5	23	10.6	30	13.8	19	8.7	0	0.0
62	32	10	31.3	17	53.1	1	3.1	2	6.3	2	6.3	0	0.0
63	69	18	26.1	36	52.2	12	17.4	2	2.9	1	1.4	0	0.0
64	28	5	17.9	20	71.4	2	7.1	1	3.6	0	0.0	0	0.0
65	43	6	14.0	29	67.4	3	7.0	4	9.3	1	2.3	0	0.0
66	118	31	26.3	61	51.7	17	14.4	5	4.2	3	2.5	1	0.8
67	173	35	20.2	82	47.4	20	11.6	17	9.8	19	11.0	0	0.0
68	262	70	26.7	86	32.8	27	10.3	32	12.2	45	17.2	2	0.8
69	124	33	26.6	37	29.8	17	13.7	17	13.7	19	15.3	1	0.8

TABLE B-4 (Continued)
Percentage Distribution of People Admitted to Public and Private Mental Hospitals by Community Area and Marital Status

C.A.	Totl.	Sgle.	%	Mar.	%	Wid.	%	Div.	%	Sep.	%	Unkn.	%
70	44	5	11.4	34	77.3	3	6.8	2	4.5	0	0.0	0	0.0
71	159	44	27.7	67	42.1	20	12.6	14	8.8	13	8.2	1	0.6
72	64	14	21.9	35	54.7	10	15.6	3	4.7	2	3.1	0	0.0
73	77	14	18.2	44	57.1	9	11.7	5	6.5	5	6.5	0	0.0
74	39	10	25.6	24	61.5	5	12.8	0	0.0	0	0.0	0	0.0
75	58	9	15.5	32	55.2	6	10.3	9	15.5	2	3.4	0	0.0
Un-known	241	90	37.3	16	6.6	19	7.9	60	24.9	43	17.8	13	5.4

176

TABLE B-5
Percentage Distribution of People
Admitted to Public and Private Mental Hospitals
by Community Area and Place of Birth

C.A.	Total	%	U.S. Born	%	Foreign Born	%	Un-known	%
City Totals	10653		5691	53.4	817	7.7	6940	65.1
1	214	100	47	22.0	14	6.5	153	71.5
2	167	100	30	18.0	5	3.0	132	79.0
3	575	100	270	47.0	44	7.6	261	45.4
4	143	100	48	33.6	5	3.5	90	62.9
5	92	100	39	42.4	7	7.6	46	50.0
6	381	100	161	42.2	23	6.0	197	51.7
7	310	100	154	49.7	43	13.9	113	36.5
8	452	100	272	60.2	47	10.4	133	29.4
9	24	100	1	4.2	2	8.3	21	87.5
10	55	100	9	16.4	3	5.4	43	78.2
11	48	100	5	10.4	3	6.2	40	83.3
12	32	100	6	18.8	3	9.4	23	71.9
13	52	100	10	19.2	2	3.8	40	76.9
14	155	100	27	17.4	13	8.4	115	74.2
15	149	100	44	29.5	9	6.0	96	64.4
16	132	100	55	41.7	10	7.6	67	50.8
17	87	100	22	25.3	10	11.5	55	63.2
18	24	100	6	25.0	1	4.2	17	70.8
19	144	100	35	24.3	11	7.6	98	68.1
20	53	100	19	35.8	3	5.7	31	58.5
21	80	100	33	41.2	6	7.5	41	51.3
22	260	100	120	46.2	31	11.9	109	41.9
23	182	100	79	43.4	13	7.1	90	49.5
24	400	100	196	49.0	98	24.5	106	26.5
25	357	100	117	32.8	30	8.4	210	58.8
26	122	100	70	57.4	12	9.8	40	32.8
27	172	100	127	73.8	18	10.5	27	15.7
28	876	100	745	85.0	69	7.9	62	7.1
29	213	100	174	81.7	8	3.8	31	14.6
30	160	100	76	47.5	16	10.0	68	42.5
31	120	100	57	47.5	22	18.3	41	34.2
32	239	100	206	86.2	8	3.3	25	10.5
33	48	100	39	81.2	1	2.1	8	16.7
34	42	100	22	52.4	5	11.9	15	35.7
35	153	100	123	80.4	2	1.3	28	18.3
36	60	100	52	86.7	1	1.7	7	11.7
37	23	100	16	69.5	0	0.0	7	30.4
38	229	100	214	93.4	0	0.0	15	6.6
39	105	100	81	77.1	2	1.9	22	21.0
40	143	100	128	89.5	3	2.1	12	8.4

TABLE B-5a
Percentage Distribution of People
Admitted to Public and Private Mental Hospitals
by Community Area and Place of Birth

C.A.	Total	%	U.S. Born	%	Foreign Born	%	Un- known	%
41	191	100	89	46.6	9	4.7	93	48.7
42	261	100	223	85.4	10	3.8	28	10.7
43	263	100	87	33.1	12	4.6	164	62.4
44	103	100	68	66.0	4	3.9	31	30.1
45	30	100	9	30.0	0	0.0	21	70.0
46	110	100	45	40.9	10	9.1	55	50.0
47	9	100	3	33.3	2	22.2	4	44.4
48	34	100	8	23.5	0	0.0	26	76.5
49	120	100	57	47.5	6	5.0	57	47.5
50	25	100	12	48.0	3	12.0	10	40.0
51	49	100	16	32.6	5	10.2	28	57.1
52	36	100	8	22.2	3	8.3	25	69.4
53	43	100	17	39.5	1	2.3	25	58.1
54	19	100	18	94.7	0	0.0	1	5.3
55	13	100	5	38.5	0	0.0	8	61.5
56	74	100	29	39.2	8	10.8	37	50.0
57	22	100	8	36.4	2	9.1	12	54.5
58	74	100	27	36.5	11	14.9	36	48.6
59	31	100	17	54.8	0	0.0	14	45.2
60	124	100	56	45.2	17	13.7	51	41.1
61	218	100	119	54.6	26	11.9	73	33.5
62	32	100	12	37.5	3	9.4	17	53.1
63	69	100	24	34.8	6	8.7	39	56.5
64	28	100	7	25.0	0	0.0	21	75.0
65	43	100	16	37.2	1	2.3	26	60.5
66	118	100	29	24.6	12	10.2	77	65.3
67	173	100	81	46.8	17	9.8	75	43.4
68	262	100	208	79.4	11	4.2	43	16.4
69	124	100	106	85.5	1	0.8	17	13.7
70	44	100	6	13.6	1	2.3	37	84.1
71	159	100	59	54.1	9	5.7	91	57.2
72	64	100	10	15.6	1	1.6	53	82.8
73	77	100	29	37.7	5	6.5	43	55.8
74	39	100	10	25.6	2	5.1	27	69.2
75	58	100	30	51.7	1	1.7	27	46.6
Un- known	241		208	86.3	15	6.2	18	7.5

TABLE B-6
Admission Rates per 100,000 Population for
Chicago People Admitted to 44 Public and Private Mental Institutions
by Diagnosis for Fiscal Year 1961

C.A.	Adult Pop. Base (1960)	Tot. (All Diagn.)	Schizo-phrenics	Schiz. First Admiss.	Manic Depress.	Senile & Arterio-sclerotics	Alcohol.	P P, P N, & P D
City To-tals	2,482,165	429.2	125.0	28.5	19.3	297.8	95.5	92.4
1	46,594	459.3	132.3	41.5	51.9	211.1	25.8	161.0
2	49,630	336.5	67.3	23.2	37.2	213.1	14.1	153.1
3	105,056	547.3	154.3	32.5	52.2	381.3	112.3	111.4
4	39,910	358.3	129.0	45.0	27.0	149.8	30.1	125.3
5	33,460	275.0	75.1	25.0	10.7	200.0	47.8	80.7
6	95,609	398.5	122.1	27.4	24.9	195.2	61.7	123.4
7	67,815	457.1	127.7	34.5	19.0	344.6	113.5	101.7
8	57,531	785.7	208.7	22.1	24.1	461.3	269.4	139.1
9	8,888	270.0	52.2	39.1	0.0	326.5	11.3	123.8
10	30,086	182.8	60.6	34.1	15.2	190.0	6.6	56.5
11	21,106	227.4	61.1	27.8	33.3	128.5	0.0	85.3
12	14,683	217.9	62.3	31.1	15.6	217.4	20.4	61.3
13	14,085	369.2	90.3	24.6	24.6	105.3	21.3	177.5
14	39,368	393.7	111.8	21.7	52.8	139.7	15.2	165.1
15	51,165	291.2	105.8	47.0	25.9	138.8	27.4	86.0
16	45,102	292.7	94.8	29.0	7.9	238.1	26.6	88.7
17	31,208	278.8	94.8	36.5	21.9	211.1	19.2	80.1

179

TABLE B-6 (Continued)
Admission Rates per 100,000 Population for Chicago People Admitted to 44 Public and Private Mental Institutions by Diagnosis for Fiscal Year 1961

C.A.	Adult Pop. Base (1960)	Tot. (All Diagn.)	Schizo-phrenics	Schiz. First Admiss.	Manic Depress.	Senile & Arterio-sclerotics	Alcohol.	P P, P N, & P D
18	9,153	262.2	103.6	25.9	25.9	139.6	0.0	43.7
19	47,353	304.1	105.0	35.0	22.5	149.6	25.3	95.0
20	16,447	322.2	100.7	36.0	21.6	354.2	30.4	73.0
21	30,009	266.6	85.8	35.1	11.7	183.1	43.3	50.0
22	70,336	369.7	117.7	26.5	19.9	229.3	75.4	81.0
23	52,892	344.1	100.5	30.6	21.8	295.2	41.6	85.1
24	98,266	407.1	133.9	29.1	18.6	340.1	85.5	66.1
25	97,744	365.2	97.1	39.3	24.6	305.5	52.2	97.2
26	31,627	385.7	114.5	21.5	17.9	325.5	98.0	66.4
27	41,825	411.2	149.4	30.9	7.7	466.4	86.1	55.0
28	80,299	1090.9	193.2	23.3	11.0	888.2	633.9	63.5
29	72,400	294.2	134.8	11.7	4.4	458.9	47.0	24.9
30	45,600	350.9	116.9	28.0	20.3	208.0	68.0	81.1
31	33,533	357.9	136.9	20.5	3.4	347.4	65.6	62.6
32	4,280	5584.1	819.0	29.2	29.2	1161.4	3808.4	233.6
33	6,260	766.8	239.6	55.3	0.0	598.8	207.7	127.8
34	10,174	412.8	203.0	22.6	0.0	382.8	68.8	19.7
35	32,186	475.4	144.9	17.2	0.0	595.4	105.6	71.5
36	13,996	428.7	179.1	15.6	0.0	868.1	92.9	35.7
37	7,305	314.9	132.8	14.8	14.8	566.0	54.8	13.7
38	57,951	393.4	152.6	9.9	7.9	520.6	65.6	31.1

TABLE B-6 (Continued)
Admission Rates per 100,000 Population for
Chicago People Admitted to 44 Public and Private Mental Institutions
by Diagnosis for Fiscal Year 1961

C.A.	Adult Pop. Base (1960)	Tot. (All Diagn.)	Schizo-phrenics	Schiz. First Admiss.	Manic Depress.	Senile & Arterio-sclerotics	Alcohol.	PP, PN, & PD
39	28,721	365.6	167.6	26.7	7.6	365.4	48.7	48.7
40	33,752	423.7	155.8	6.8	6.8	473.3	83.0	44.4
41	36,050	529.8	188.4	48.7	32.5	208.7	83.2	180.3
42	57,704	452.3	180.7	13.3	15.2	527.5	76.3	55.5
43	59,953	438.7	123.8	35.1	37.2	130.4	85.1	151.8
44	32,296	318.9	118.8	34.9	21.0	299.6	43.3	46.4
45	9,384	319.7	75.4	37.7	37.7	279.8	32.0	117.2
46	36,112	304.6	101.9	31.8	22.3	297.9	44.3	77.5
47	2,489	361.6	186.6	93.3	0.0	289.9	40.1	40.2
48	13,589	250.2	73.8	16.4	24.6	142.8	7.4	103.0
49	43,151	278.1	78.6	16.3	35.2	192.0	32.4	83.4
50	6,134	407.6	93.1	0.0	0.0	262.8	114.1	48.9
51	12,347	396.7	125.4	35.8	53.7	338.7	32.4	145.8
52	16,791	214.4	67.0	26.8	20.1	107.4	23.8	71.5
53	24,799	173.4	50.8	23.1	23.1	95.6	24.2	48.4
54	4,941	384.5	194.2	0.0	21.6	325.7	0.0	60.7
55	6,244	208.2	89.8	35.9	35.9	0.0	16.0	64.1
56	26,273	281.7	73.9	8.2	12.3	469.0	30.4	95.2
57	7,811	281.7	104.4	14.9	44.7	0.0	25.6	102.4
58	28,249	261.9	86.3	28.8	8.2	152.8	42.5	60.2
59	12,135	255.5	76.0	9.5	0.0	0.0	41.2	82.4

TABLE B-6 (Continued)
Admission Rates per 100,000 Population for
Chicago People Admitted to 44 Public and Private Mental Institutions
by Diagnosis for Fiscal Year 1961

C.A.	Adult Pop. Base (1960)	Tot. (All Diagn.)	Schizo-phrenics	Schiz. First Admiss.	Manic Depress.	Senile & Arterio-sclerotics	Alcohol.	P P, P N, & P D
60	29,111	426.0	146.9	55.6	23.8	255.1	82.4	89.3
61	47,276	461.1	150.0	33.9	24.2	235.9	116.3	107.9
62	10,464	305.8	95.3	31.8	21.2	196.7	28.7	86.0
63	21,998	313.7	102.1	37.6	26.9	265.5	45.5	95.5
64	12,801	218.7	100.8	58.8	16.8	223.0	31.2	39.1
65	19,437	221.2	91.8	51.6	0.0	49.7	25.7	56.6
66	40,972	288.0	77.9	28.9	17.3	221.1	41.5	104.9
67	42,601	406.1	132.2	38.6	33.1	333.7	84.5	98.6
68	63,352	415.1	161.9	22.9	7.0	368.2	112.1	50.5
69	45,310	273.7	115.0	17.1	4.9	405.9	35.3	35.3
70	13,350	329.6	101.3	42.2	25.3	199.2	22.5	142.3
71	46,535	341.7	60.3	21.0	31.4	263.1	75.2	103.1
72	18,024	355.1	79.7	59.8	33.2	404.6	11.1	149.8
73	21,813	353.0	96.7	26.9	26.9	250.5	50.4	114.6
74	14,433	270.2	68.2	15.2	15.2	561.8	13.9	83.1
75	19,381	299.3	79.2	18.3	24.4	236.4	31.0	87.7

TABLE B-7
Number of First Admissions (City of Chicago Residents)
to 44 Public and Private Mental Institutions
by Diagnosis for Fiscal Year 1961

C.A.	Adult Population Base (1960)	Total	Schizo-phrenics	Manic Depres-sives	Senile & Arterio-sclerotics	Alcohol-ics	PP, PN PD
City Totals	2,482,165	3,431	635	197	131	634	1,351
1	46,594	97	16	11	5	5	47
2	49,630	81	10	8	2	2	50
3	105,056	189	28	17	8	43	66
4	39,910	60	15	4	4	3	29
5	33,460	37	7	1	2	5	16
6	95,609	149	22	12	6	23	73
7	67,815	84	20	5	5	17	29
8	57,531	119	11	1	5	47	39
9	8,888	18	3	0	2	0	10
10	30,086	27	9	2	1	0	12
11	21,106	30	5	5	1	0	14
12	14,683	19	4	1	2	2	6
13	14,085	25	3	1	1	0	16
14	39,368	64	7	4	2	2	43
15	51,165	70	20	3	0	4	29
16	45,102	53	11	1	3	2	28
17	31,208	40	10	1	2	4	19
18	9,153	7	2	0	0	0	3
19	47,353	73	14	5	2	6	31

TABLE B-7 (Continued)
Number of First Admissions (City of Chicago Residents) to 44 Public and Private Mental Institutions by Diagnosis for Fiscal Year 1961

C.A.	Adult Population Base (1960)	Total	Schizo-phrenics	Manic Depres-sives	Senile & Arterio-sclerotics	Alcohol-ics	PP, PN PD
20	16,447	25	5	0	7	1	8
21	30,009	33	9	0	2	3	12
22	70,336	89	16	4	4	16	38
23	52,892	71	14	4	3	6	29
24	98,266	110	25	4	5	23	32
25	97,744	153	32	7	10	18	62
26	31,627	34	6	4	1	7	11
27	41,825	33	12	2	1	6	9
28	80,299	213	17	3	4	154	27
29	72,400	27	8	1	3	3	7
30	45,600	50	11	5	1	7	20
31	33,533	35	6	0	1	8	12
32	4,280	58	1	0	1	47	4
33	6,260	13	3	0	0	6	3
34	10,174	8	2	0	1	1	2
35	32,186	26	5	0	1	4	11
36	13,996	6	2	0	1	1	1
37	7,305	2	1	0	0	0	1
38	57,951	22	5	0	1	6	7
39	28,721	18	7	2	1	1	6
40	33,752	11	2	0	1	0	5

TABLE B-7 (Continued)
Number of First Admissions (City of Chicago Residents)
to 44 Public and Private Mental Institutions
by Diagnosis for Fiscal Year 1961

C.A.	Adult Population Base (1960)	Total	Schizo-phrenics	Manic Depres-sives	Senile & Arterio-sclerotics	Alcohol-ics	PP, PN PD
41	36,050	71	15	3	0	9	38
42	57,704	38	7	3	0	5	15
43	59,953	105	17	8	1	17	50
44	32,296	28	10	1	1	3	9
45	9,384	17	3	2	1	1	9
46	36,112	41	11	2	3	5	16
47	2,489	3	2	0	0	0	1
48	13,589	14	2	1	0	1	8
49	43,151	49	6	10	3	7	19
50	6,134	6	0	0	0	4	1
51	12,347	21	4	2	0	2	12
52	16,791	17	4	1	0	2	8
53	24,799	21	5	3	1	3	7
54	4,941	2	0	1	0	0	1
55	6,244	4	2	0	0	0	2
56	26,273	27	2	2	0	2	17
57	7,811	8	1	1	0	0	4
58	28,249	24	7	1	0	3	9
59	12,135	13	1	0	0	2	8
60	29,111	52	14	3	1	10	17
61	47,276	69	14	4	1	19	27

TABLE B-7 (Continued)
Number of First Admissions (City of Chicago Residents)
to 44 Public and Private Mental Institutions
by Diagnosis for Fiscal Year 1961

C.A.	Adult Population Base (1960)	Total	Schizo- phrenics	Manic Depres- sives	Senile & Arterio- sclerotics	Alcohol- ics	PP, PN PD
62	10,464	14	3	1	0	1	5
63	21,998	26	7	2	0	3	12
64	12,801	17	7	1	1	1	4
65	19,437	20	9	0	0	1	7
66	40,972	58	10	5	1	4	32
67	42,601	63	14	4	4	10	28
68	63,352	52	13	0	1	16	17
69	45,310	24	7	1	0	1	10
70	13,350	29	5	3	1	1	17
71	46,535	68	8	5	5	12	27
72	18,024	32	9	3	3	0	14
73	21,813	29	5	3	0	5	12
74	14,433	19	2	0	0	0	10
75	19,381	21	3	3	1	1	11

TABLE B-8
First Admission Rates per 100,000
Age Specific Populations to
44 Public and Private Mental Institutions
by Diagnosis for Fiscal Year 1961.

C.A.	Total	Schizo-phrenics	Manic Depres-sives	Senile & Arterio-sclerotics	Alcohol-ics	P P, P N, & P D
City Rates	138.2	28.4	7.9	37.8	25.5	54.4
1	20.2	41.5	23.6	062.1	10.7	100.9
2	163.2	23.2	16.1	30.5	4.0	100.7
3	179.9	32.5	16.2	42.4	40.9	62.8
4	150.3	45.0	10.0	59.9	7.5	72.7
5	110.6	25.0	3.0	36.4	14.9	47.8
6	155.8	27.4	12.6	39.0	24.1	76.4
7	123.9	34.5	7.4	50.7	25.1	42.8
8	206.8	22.1	1.7	65.0	81.7	67.8
9	202.5	39.1	0.0	163.3	0.0	112.5
10	89.7	34.1	6.6	27.1	0.0	39.9
11	142.1	27.8	23.7	32.1	0.0	66.3
12	129.4	31.1	6.8	108.7	13.6	40.9
13	177.5	24.6	7.1	52.6	0.0	113.6
14	162.6	21.7	10.2	27.9	5.1	109.2
15	136.8	47.0	5.9	0.0	7.8	56.7
16	117.5	29.0	2.2	42.0	4.4	62.1
17	128.2	36.5	3.2	52.8	12.8	60.9
18	76.5	25.9	0.0	0.0	0.0	32.8
19	154.2	35.0	10.6	27.2	12.7	65.5
20	152.0	36.0	0.0	275.5	6.1	48.6
21	110.0	35.1	0.0	45.8	10.0	40.0
22	126.5	26.5	5.7	39.9	22.7	31.3
23	134.2	30.6	7.6	42.2	11.3	54.8
24	111.9	29.1	4.1	40.5	23.4	32.6
25	156.5	39.3	7.2	61.1	18.4	63.4
26	107.5	21.5	12.6	27.1	22.1	34.8
27	78.9	30.9	4.8	33.3	14.3	21.5
28	265.3	23.3	3.7	54.7	191.8	33.6
29	37.3	11.7	1.4	72.5	4.1	9.7
30	109.6	28.0	11.0	16.0	15.4	43.9
31	104.4	20.5	0.0	23.2	23.9	35.8
32	1355.1	29.2	0.0	116.1	1098.1	93.5
33	207.7	55.3	0.0	0.0	95.8	47.9
34	78.6	22.6	0.0	76.6	9.8	19.7
35	80.8	17.2	0.0	31.3	12.4	34.2
36	42.9	15.6	0.0	86.8	7.1	7.1
37	27.4	14.8	0.0	0.0	0.0	13.7
38	38.0	9.9	0.0	13.4	10.4	12.1

TABLE B-8 (Continued)
First Admission Rates per 100,000
Age Specific Populations to
44 Public and Private Mental Institutions
by Diagnosis for Fiscal Year 1961.

C.A.	Total	Schizo-phrenics	Manic Depres-sives	Senile & Arterio-sclerotics	Alcohol-ics	P P, P N, & P D
39	62.7	26.7	7.0	40.6	3.5	20.9
40	32.6	6.8	0.0	23.7	0.0	14.8
41	196.9	48.7	8.9	0.0	25.0	105.4
42	65.9	13.3	5.2	0.0	8.7	26.0
43	175.1	35.1	13.3	8.7	28.4	83.4
44	86.7	34.9	3.1	27.2	9.3	27.9
45	181.2	37.7	21.3	69.9	10.7	95.9
46	113.5	31.8	5.5	63.8	13.8	44.3
47	120.5	93.3	0.0	0.0	0.0	40.2
48	103.0	16.4	7.4	0.0	7.4	58.9
49	113.6	16.3	23.2	48.0	16.2	44.0
50	97.8	0.0	0.0	0.0	65.2	16.3
51	170.0	35.8	16.2	0.0	16.2	97.2
52	101.2	26.8	6.0	0.0	11.9	47.6
53	84.7	23.1	12.1	31.9	12.1	28.2
54	40.5	0.0	20.2	0.0	0.0	20.2
55	64.1	35.9	0.0	0.0	0.0	32.0
56	102.8	8.2	7.6	0.0	7.6	64.7
57	102.4	14.9	12.8	0.0	0.0	51.2
58	85.0	28.8	3.5	0.0	10.6	31.9
59	107.1	9.5	0.0	0.0	16.5	65.9
60	178.6	55.6	10.3	25.5	34.4	58.4
61	146.0	33.9	8.5	16.9	40.2	57.1
62	133.8	31.8	9.6	0.0	9.6	47.8
63	118.2	37.6	9.1	0.0	13.6	54.6
64	132.8	58.8	7.8	111.5	7.8	31.2
65	102.9	51.6	0.0	0.0	5.1	36.0
66	141.6	28.9	12.2	15.8	9.8	78.1
67	147.9	38.6	9.4	63.6	23.5	67.7
68	82.1	22.9	0.0	15.3	25.3	26.8
69	53.0	17.1	2.2	0.0	2.2	22.1
70	217.2	42.2	22.5	66.4	7.5	127.3
71	146.1	21.0	10.7	59.8	25.8	58.0
72	177.5	59.8	16.6	101.2	0.0	77.7
73	132.9	26.9	13.8	0.0	22.9	55.0
74	131.6	15.2	0.0	0.0	0.0	69.3
75	108.4	18.3	15.5	33.8	5.2	56.8

TABLE B-9

Number of Readmissions (City of Chicago Residents)
to 44 Public and Private Mental Institutions
by Diagnosis for Fiscal Year 1961.

C.A.	Adult Population Base (1960)	Total	Schizo- phrenics	Manic Depres- sives	Senile & Arterio- sclerotics	Alcohol- ics	PP, PN, & PD
City Totals	2,482,165	5,796	2,108	277	833	1,599	929
1	46,594	91	35	9	12	7	28
2	49,630	70	19	8	12	5	26
3	105,056	323	105	28	64	75	51
4	39,910	69	28	5	6	9	21
5	33,460	47	14	2	9	11	11
6	95,609	189	76	8	24	36	45
7	67,815	189	54	6	29	60	40
8	57,531	283	93	11	30	108	41
9	8,888	5	1	0	2	1	1
10	30,086	22	7	2	6	2	5
11	21,106	14	6	1	3	0	4
12	14,683	11	4	1	2	1	3
13	14,085	23	8	2	1	3	9
14	39,368	76	29	13	8	4	22
15	51,165	70	25	8	12	10	15
16	45,102	63	25	2	14	10	12
17	31,208	35	16	5	6	2	6
18	9,153	11	6	2	2	0	1
19	47,353	61	28	4	9	6	14

TABLE B-9 (Continued)
Number of Readmissions (City of Chicago Residents) to 44 Public and Private Mental Institutions by Diagnosis for Fiscal Year 1961.

C.A.	Adult Population Base (1960)	Total	Schizo-phrenics	Manic Depres-sives	Senile & Arterio-sclerotics	Alcohol-ics	PP, PN, & PD
20	16,447	22	9	3	2	4	4
21	30,009	35	13	3	6	10	3
22	70,336	138	55	8	19	37	19
23	52,892	89	32	6	19	16	16
24	98,266	233	90	12	37	61	33
25	97,744	166	47	13	40	33	33
26	31,627	72	26	1	11	24	10
27	41,825	104	46	1	13	30	14
28	80,299	569	124	5	61	355	24
29	72,400	144	84	2	16	31	11
30	45,600	91	35	3	12	24	17
31	33,533	72	34	1	14	14	9
32	4,280	159	27	1	9	116	6
33	6,260	27	10	0	5	7	5
34	10,174	26	16	0	4	6	0
35	32,186	97	37	0	18	30	12
36	13,996	46	21	0	9	12	4
37	7,305	16	8	1	3	4	0
38	57,951	157	72	4	38	32	11
39	28,721	66	37	0	8	13	8
40	33,752	103	44	2	19	28	10

TABLE B-9 (Continued)
Number of Readmissions (City of Chicago Residents)
to 44 Public and Private Mental Institutions
by Diagnosis for Fiscal Year 1961.

C.A.	Adult Population Base (1960)	Total	Schizo-phrenics	Manic Depres-sives	Senile & Arterio-sclerotics	Alcohol-ics	PP, PN, & PD
41	36,050	109	43	7	11	21	27
42	57,704	176	88	5	27	39	17
43	59,953	142	43	10	14	34	41
44	32,296	56	24	5	10	11	6
45	9,384	11	3	1	3	2	2
46	36,112	60	21	5	11	11	12
47	2,489	4	2	0	1	1	0
48	13,589	17	7	2	1	0	6
49	43,151	59	23	3	2	7	17
50	6,134	12	5	0	9	3	2
51	12,347	26	10	4	2	2	6
52	16,791	16	6	2	4	2	4
53	24,799	18	6	2	2	3	5
54	4,941	12	9	0	1	0	2
55	6,244	8	3	2	0	1	2
56	26,273	40	16	1	9	6	8
57	7,811	14	6	2	0	2	4
58	28,249	38	14	1	6	9	8
59	12,135	12	7	0	0	3	2
60	29,111	58	23	3	9	14	9
61	47,276	127	48	6	13	36	24

TABLE B-9 (Continued)
Number of Readmissions (City of Chicago Residents) to 44 Public and Private Mental Institutions by Diagnosis for Fiscal Year 1961.

C.A.	Adult Population Base (1960)	Total	Schizo-phrenics	Manic Depres-sives	Senile & Arterio-sclerotics	Alcohol-ics	PP, PN, & PD
62	10,464	15	6	1	2	2	4
63	21,998	40	12	3	9	7	9
64	12,801	11	5	1	1	3	1
65	19,437	16	7	0	1	4	4
66	40,972	55	17	1	13	13	11
67	42,601	89	34	8	17	16	14
68	63,352	176	79	4	23	55	15
69	45,310	80	40	1	18	15	6
70	13,350	13	7	0	2	2	2
71	46,535	83	15	7	17	23	21
72	18,024	29	3	2	9	2	13
73	21,813	42	13	2	8	6	13
74	14,433	20	7	2	7	2	2
75	19,381	28	10	1	6	5	6

TABLE B-10
Readmission Rates per 100,000
Age Specific Populations to 44 Public
and Private Mental Institutions
by Diagnosis for Fiscal Year 1961.

C.A.	Total	Schizo-phrenics	Manic Depres-sives	Senile & Arterio-sclerotics	Alcohol-ics	PP, PN, & PD
City Rates	233.5	84.9	11.2	35.6	64.4	37.4
1	195.3	90.8	19.3	149.0	15.0	60.1
2	141.0	44.1	16.1	182.7	10.1	52.4
3	307.5	121.9	26.7	339.0	71.4	48.6
4	172.9	84.0	12.5	89.9	22.6	52.6
5	140.5	50.1	6.0	163.6	32.9	32.9
6	197.7	94.7	8.4	156.2	37.7	47.1
7	278.7	93.2	8.9	293.9	88.5	59.0
8	491.9	186.6	19.1	390.2	187.7	71.3
9	56.3	13.1	0.0	163.3	11.3	11.3
10	73.1	26.5	6.7	162.8	6.7	16.6
11	66.3	33.3	4.7	96.4	0.0	19.0
12	74.9	31.2	6.8	108.7	6.8	20.4
13	163.3	65.7	14.2	52.6	21.3	63.9
14	193.1	90.0	33.0	111.8	10.2	55.9
15	136.8	58.8	15.6	138.8	19.6	29.3
16	139.7	65.9	4.4	196.1	22.2	26.6
17	112.2	58.4	16.0	158.3	6.4	19.2
18	120.2	77.7	21.9	139.6	0.0	10.9
19	128.8	70.0	8.5	122.4	12.7	29.6
20	133.8	64.7	18.2	78.7	24.3	24.3
21	116.6	50.7	10.0	137.3	33.3	10.0
22	196.2	91.2	11.4	189.5	52.6	27.0
23	168.3	69.9	11.3	267.1	30.3	30.3
24	237.1	104.8	12.2	299.6	62.1	33.6
25	169.8	57.8	13.3	244.4	33.8	33.8
26	227.7	93.1	3.2	298.4	75.9	31.6
27	248.7	118.5	2.4	433.1	71.8	33.5
28	708.6	169.9	6.2	833.6	442.1	29.9
29	198.9	123.1	2.8	386.5	42.8	15.2
30	199.6	88.9	6.6	192.0	52.6	37.3
31	214.7	116.4	3.0	324.2	41.8	26.8
32	3715.0	789.7	23.4	1045.3	2710.3	140.2
33	431.3	184.3	0.0	598.8	111.8	79.9
34	255.6	180.4	0.0	306.3	59.0	0.0
35	301.4	127.6	0.0	564.1	93.2	37.3
36	328.7	163.5	0.0	781.3	85.7	28.6
37	219.0	118.1	13.7	566.0	54.8	0.0

TABLE B-10 (Continued)
Readmission Rates per 100,000
Age Specific Populations to 44 Public
and Private Mental Institutions
by Diagnosis for Fiscal Year 1961.

C.A.	Total	Schizo- phrenics	Manic Depres- sives	Senile & Arterio- sclerotics	Alcohol- ics	PP, PN, & PD
38	270.9	142.7	6.9	507.3	55.2	19.0
39	229.8	140.9	0.0	324.8	45.3	27.9
40	305.2	149.0	5.9	449.6	83.0	29.6
41	302.4	139.7	19.4	208.7	58.3	74.9
42	305.0	167.3	8.7	527.6	67.6	29.5
43	236.9	88.8	16.7	121.7	56.7	68.4
44	173.4	83.8	15.5	272.4	34.1	18.6
45	117.2	37.7	10.7	209.8	21.3	21.3
46	166.1	66.9	13.9	234.1	30.5	33.2
47	160.7	93.3	0.0	46.6	40.2	0.0
48	125.1	57.4	14.7	142.8	0.0	44.2
49	136.7	62.3	7.0	144.0	16.2	39.4
50	195.6	93.1	0.0	262.8	49.9	32.6
51	210.6	89.6	32.4	338.7	16.2	48.6
52	95.3	40.2	11.9	107.4	11.9	23.8
53	72.6	27.7	8.1	63.7	12.1	20.2
54	242.9	194.2	0.0	325.7	0.0	40.5
55	128.1	53.9	32.0	0.0	16.0	32.0
56	152.2	65.7	3.8	469.0	22.8	30.5
57	179.2	89.5	25.6	0.0	25.6	51.2
58	134.5	57.6	3.5	152.8	31.9	28.3
59	98.9	66.5	0.0	0.0	24.7	16.5
60	199.2	91.3	10.3	229.6	48.1	30.9
61	268.6	116.1	12.7	219.0	76.2	50.8
62	143.3	63.5	9.6	196.7	19.1	38.2
63	181.8	64.5	13.6	265.5	31.8	40.9
64	85.9	42.0	7.8	111.5	23.4	7.8
65	82.3	40.2	0.0	49.7	20.6	20.6
66	134.2	49.1	2.4	205.3	31.7	26.9
67	208.9	93.7	18.8	270.1	37.6	32.9
68	277.8	139.0	6.3	352.8	86.8	23.7
69	176.6	97.9	2.2	406.0	33.1	13.2
70	97.4	59.1	0.0	132.8	15.0	15.0
71	178.4	39.3	15.0	203.3	49.4	45.1
72	160.9	19.9	11.1	303.4	11.1	72.1
73	192.5	69.8	9.2	250.5	27.5	59.6
74	138.6	53.1	13.9	561.8	13.9	13.9
75	144.5	60.9	5.2	202.6	25.8	31.0

TABLE B-11

Number of People Admitted (City of Chicago Residents) to 44 Public and Private Mental Institutions by Type of Institution and Community Area for Fiscal Year 1961

	Adult Population Base (1960)	Number of People Admitted to:				Admission Rate/100,000 Adult Population			
		All Facilities	State Hosp.	Psych. Wards of Gen. Hosp.	Private Mental Hosp.	All Facilities	State Hosp.	Psych. Wards of Gen. Hosp.	Private Mental Hosp.
City Totals	2,482,165	10,653	6,725	2,404	1,524	429.2	270.9	96.9	61.4
1	46,594	214	64	91	59	459.3	137.4	195.3	126.6
2	49,630	167	36	89	42	336.5	72.9	179.3	84.6
3	105,056	575	332	139	104	547.3	316.0	132.3	99.0
4	39,910	143	55	48	40	358.3	137.8	120.3	100.2
5	33,460	92	50	23	19	275.0	149.4	68.7	56.8
6	95,609	381	187	117	77	398.5	195.6	122.4	80.5
7	67,815	310	208	59	43	457.1	306.7	87.0	63.4
8	57,531	452	328	86	38	785.7	570.1	149.5	66.1
9	8,888	24	4	10	10	270.0	45.0	112.5	112.5
10	30,086	55	12	18	25	182.8	39.9	59.8	83.1
11	21,106	48	8	15	25	227.4	37.9	71.1	118.4
12	14,683	32	9	16	7	217.9	61.3	109.0	47.7
13	14,085	52	12	27	13	369.2	85.2	191.7	92.3
14	39,368	155	44	71	40	393.7	111.8	180.3	101.6

TABLE B-11 (Continued)
Number of People Admitted (City of Chicago Residents) to 44 Public and Private Mental Institutions by Type of Institution and Community Area for Fiscal Year 1961

	Adult Popu-lation Base (1960)	Number of People Admitted to:				Admission Rate/100,000 Adult Population			
		All Facil-ities	State Hosp.	Psych. Wards of Gen. Hosp.	Private Mental Hosp.	All Facil-ities	State Hosp.	Psych. Wards of Gen. Hosp.	Private Mental Hosp.
15	51,165	149	55	46	48	291.2	107.5	89.9	93.8
16	45,102	132	66	29	37	292.7	146.3	64.3	82.0
17	31,208	87	32	29	26	278.8	102.5	92.9	83.3
18	9,153	24	9	7	8	262.2	98.3	76.5	87.4
19	47,353	144	48	49	47	304.1	101.4	103.5	99.3
20	16,447	53	22	18	13	322.2	322.2	109.4	79.0
21	30,009	80	39	12	29	266.6	130.0	40.0	96.6
22	70,336	260	158	42	60	369.7	224.6	59.7	85.3
23	52,892	182	95	49	38	344.1	179.6	92.6	71.8
24	98,266	400	302	29	69	407.1	307.3	29.5	70.2
25	97,744	357	149	144	64	365.2	152.4	147.3	65.5
26	31,627	122	84	27	11	385.7	265.6	85.4	34.8
27	41,825	172	153	12	7	411.2	365.8	28.7	16.7
28	80,299	876	833	31	12	1090.9	1037.4	38.6	14.9
29	72,400	213	189	15	9	294.2	261.0	20.7	12.4
30	45,600	160	93	31	36	350.9	203.9	68.0	78.9

TABLE B-11 (Continued)
Number of People Admitted (City of Chicago Residents)
to 44 Public and Private Mental Institutions
by Type of Institution and Community Area for Fiscal Year 1961

	Adult Popu- lation Base (1960)	Number of People Admitted to:				Admission Rate/100,000 Adult Population			
		All Facil- ities	State Hosp.	Psych. Wards of Gen. Hosp.	Private Mental Hosp.	All Facil- ities	State Hosp.	Psych. Wards of Gen. Hosp.	Private Mental Hosp.
31	33,533	120	81	22	17	357.9	241.6	65.6	50.7
32	4,289	239	222	8	9	5584.1	5186.9	186.9	210.3
33	6,260	48	42	2	4	766.7	670.9	31.9	63.9
34	10,174	42	32	7	3	412.8	314.5	68.8	29.5
35	32,186	153	130	16	7	475.4	403.9	49.7	21.7
36	13,996	60	57	2	1	428.7	407.3	14.3	7.1
37	7,305	23	20	1	2	314.9	273.8	13.7	27.4
38	57,951	228	220	6	2	393.4	379.6	10.4	3.5
39	28,721	105	84	18	3	365.6	292.5	62.7	10.4
40	33,752	143	136	5	2	423.7	402.9	14.8	5.9
41	36,050	191	101	72	18	529.8	280.2	199.7	49.9
42	57,704	261	244	12	5	452.3	422.8	20.8	8.7
43	59,953	263	103	122	38	438.7	171.8	203.5	63.4
44	32,296	103	75	19	9	318.9	233.2	58.8	27.9
45	9,384	30	9	14	7	319.7	95.9	149.2	74.6

TABLE B-11 (Continued)
Number of People Admitted (City of Chicago Residents)
to 44 Public and Private Mental Institutions
by Type of Institution and Community Area for Fiscal Year 1961

	Adult Population Base (1960)	Number of People Admitted to:				Admission Rate/100,000 Adult Population			
		All Facilities	State Hosp.	Psych. Wards of Gen. Hosp.	Private Mental Hosp.	All Facilities	State Hosp.	Psych. Wards of Gen. Hosp.	Private Mental Hosp.
46	36,112	110	57	27	26	304.6	157.8	74.8	72.0
47	2,489	9	5	2	2	361.6	200.9	80.4	80.4
48	13,589	34	9	18	7	250.2	66.2	132.5	51.5
49	43,151	120	64	33	23	278.1	148.3	76.5	53.3
50	6,134	25	15	7	3	407.6	244.5	114.1	48.9
51	12,347	49	21	15	13	396.9	170.1	121.5	105.3
52	16,791	36	12	12	12	214.4	71.5	71.5	71.5
53	24,799	43	20	14	9	173.4	80.6	56.5	36.3
54	4,941	19	19	0	0	384.5	384.5	0.0	0.0
55	6,244	13	5	4	4	208.2	80.1	64.1	64.1
56	26,273	74	37	20	17	281.7	140.8	76.1	64.7
57	7,811	22	10	9	3	281.7	128.0	115.2	38.4
58	28,249	74	40	22	12	262.0	141.6	77.9	42.5
59	12,135	31	17	8	6	255.5	140.1	65.9	49.4
60	29,111	124	75	28	21	426.0	257.6	96.2	72.1

TABLE B-11 (Continued)
Number of People Admitted (City of Chicago Residents)
to 44 Public and Private Mental Institutions
by Type of Institution and Community Area for Fiscal Year 1961

	Number of People Admitted to:				Admission Rate/100,000 Adult Population			
Adult Popu- lation Base (1960)	All Facil- ities	State Hosp.	Psych. Wards of Gen. Hosp.	Private Mental Hosp.	All Facil- ities	State Hosp.	Psych. Wards of Gen. Hosp.	Private Mental Hosp.
47,276	218	145	46	27	461.1	306.7	97.3	57.1
10,464	32	15	12	5	305.8	143.3	114.7	47.8
21,998	69	30	25	14	313.7	136.4	113.6	63.6
12,801	28	7	16	5	218.7	54.7	125.0	39.1
19,437	43	17	19	8	221.2	87.5	97.8	41.2
40,972	118	42	54	22	288.0	102.5	131.8	53.7
42,601	173	98	54	21	406.1	230.0	126.8	49.3
63,352	263	226	25	12	415.1	356.7	39.5	18.9
45,310	124	109	11	4	273.7	240.6	24.3	8.8
13,350	44	7	32	4	329.6	52.4	239.7	30.0
46,535	159	68	71	20	341.7	146.1	152.6	43.0
18,024	64	11	40	13	355.1	61.0	221.9	72.1
21,813	77	34	29	14	353.0	155.9	132.9	64.2
14,433	39	12	20	7	270.2	83.1	138.6	48.5
19,381	58	32	22	4	299.3	165.1	113.5	20.6

Row labels (left margin): 61, 62, 63, 64, 65, 66, 67, 68, 69, 70, 71, 72, 73, 74, 75

TABLE B-12
Number of First Admissions (City of Chicago Residents)
to 44 Public and Private Mental Institutions
by Type of Institution and Community Area for Fiscal Year 1961

C.A.	Adult Population Base (1960)	Number of First Admissions to:				First Admission Rate/100,000 Adult Population			
		All Facilities	State Hosp.	Psych. Wards of Gen. Hosp.	Private Mental Hosp.	All Facilities	State Hosp.	Psych. Wards of Gen. Hosp.	Private Mental Hosp.
City Totals	2,482,165	3,431	951	1,520	960	138.2	38.3	61.2	38.7
1	46,594	97	5	59	33	208.2	10.7	126.6	70.8
2	49,630	81	2	53	26	163.2	4.0	106.8	52.4
3	105,056	189	55	81	53	179.9	52.4	77.1	50.4
4	39,910	60	7	29	24	150.3	17.5	72.7	60.1
5	33,460	37	10	15	12	110.6	29.9	44.8	35.9
6	95,609	149	32	75	42	155.8	33.5	78.4	43.9
7	67,815	84	22	38	24	123.9	32.4	56.0	35.4
8	57,531	119	49	53	17	206.8	85.2	92.1	29.5
9	8,888	18	2	9	7	202.5	22.5	101.3	78.8
10	30,086	27	2	13	12	89.7	6.6	43.2	39.9
11	21,106	30	0	12	18	142.1	0.0	56.9	85.3
12	14,683	19	3	9	7	129.4	20.4	61.3	47.7
13	14,085	25	3	16	6	177.5	21.3	113.6	42.6
14	39,368	64	4	34	26	162.6	10.2	86.4	66.0

TABLE B-12 (Continued)
Number of First Admissions (City of Chicago Residents) to 44 Public and Private Mental Institutions by Type of Institution and Community Area for Fiscal Year 1961

C.A.	Adult Population Base (1960)	Number of First Admissions to:				First Admission Rate/100,000 Adult Population			
		All Facilities	State Hosp.	Psych. Wards of Gen. Hosp.	Private Mental Hosp.	All Facilities	State Hosp.	Psych. Wards of Gen. Hosp.	Private Mental Hosp.
15	51,165	70	6	30	34	136.8	11.7	58.6	66.5
16	45,102	53	4	23	26	117.5	9.0	51.0	57.6
17	31,208	40	6	16	18	128.2	19.2	51.3	57.7
18	9,153	7	0	4	3	76.5	0.0	43.7	32.8
19	47,353	73	10	31	32	154.2	21.1	65.5	67.6
20	16,447	25	4	13	8	152.0	24.3	79.0	48.6
21	30,009	33	3	8	22	110.0	10.0	26.7	73.3
22	70,336	89	21	30	38	126.5	29.9	42.7	54.0
23	52,892	71	17	32	22	134.2	32.1	60.5	41.6
24	98,266	110	45	21	44	111.9	45.8	21.4	44.8
25	97,744	153	24	84	45	156.5	24.6	85.9	46.0
26	31,627	34	11	15	8	107.5	34.8	47.4	25.3
27	41,825	33	17	9	7	78.9	40.6	21.5	16.7
28	80,299	213	176	27	10	265.3	219.2	33.6	12.5
29	72,400	27	8	11	8	37.3	11.0	15.2	11.0

TABLE B-12 (Continued)
Number of First Admissions (City of Chicago Residents) to 44 Public and Private Mental Institutions by Type of Institution and Community Area for Fiscal Year 1961

C.A.	Adult Population Base (1960)	Number of First Admissions to:				First Admission Rate/100,000 Adult Population			
		All Facilities	State Hosp.	Psych. Wards of Gen. Hosp.	Private Mental Hosp.	All Facilities	State Hosp.	Psych. Wards of Gen. Hosp.	Private Mental Hosp.
30	45,600	50	7	19	24	109.6	15.4	41.7	52.6
31	33,533	35	9	12	14	104.4	26.8	35.8	41.7
32	4,280	58	51	3	4	1355.1	1191.6	70.1	93.5
33	6,260	13	7	2	4	207.7	111.8	31.9	63.9
34	10,174	8	3	4	1	78.6	29.5	39.3	9.8
35	32,186	26	6	14	6	80.8	18.6	43.5	18.6
36	13,996	6	3	2	1	42.9	21.4	14.3	7.1
37	7,305	2	1	0	1	27.4	13.7	0.0	13.7
38	57,951	22	15	5	2	38.0	25.9	8.6	3.5
39	28,721	18	4	12	2	62.7	13.9	41.8	7.0
40	33,752	11	6	4	1	32.6	17.8	11.9	3.0
41	36,050	71	11	48	12	196.9	30.5	133.1	33.3
42	57,704	38	25	10	3	65.9	43.3	17.3	5.2
43	59,953	105	14	69	22	175.1	23.4	115.1	36.7
44	32,296	28	11	13	4	86.7	34.1	40.3	12.4

TABLE B-12 (Continued)
Number of First Admissions (City of Chicago Residents)
to 44 Public and Private Mental Institutions
by Type of Institution and Community Area for Fiscal Year 1961

C.A.	Adult Population Base (1960)	Number of First Admissions to:				First Admission Rate/100,000 Adult Population			
		All Facilities	State Hosp.	Psych. Wards of Gen. Hosp.	Private Mental Hosp.	All Facilities	State Hosp.	Psych. Wards of Gen. Hosp.	Private Mental Hosp.
45	9,384	17	2	10	5	181.2	21.3	106.6	53.3
46	36,112	41	8	17	16	113.5	22.2	47.1	44.3
47	2,489	3	0	2	1	120.5	0.0	80.4	40.2
48	13,589	14	0	10	4	103.0	0.0	73.6	29.4
49	43,151	49	13	19	17	113.6	30.1	44.0	39.4
50	6,134	6	4	2	0	97.8	65.2	32.6	0.0
51	12,347	21	2	10	9	170.1	16.2	81.0	72.9
52	16,791	17	2	4	11	101.2	11.9	23.8	65.5
53	24,799	21	3	10	8	84.7	12.1	40.3	32.3
54	4,941	2	2	0	0	40.5	40.5	0.0	0.0
55	6,244	4	1	2	1	64.1	16.0	32.0	16.0
56	26,273	27	3	11	13	102.8	11.4	41.9	49.5
57	7,811	8	2	5	1	102.4	25.6	64.0	12.8
58	28,249	24	3	13	8	85.0	10.6	46.0	28.3
59	12,135	13	1	7	5	107.1	8.2	57.7	41.2

TABLE B-12 (Continued)
Number of First Admissions (City of Chicago Residents) to 44 Public and Private Mental Institutions by Type of Institution and Community Area for Fiscal Year 1961

C.A.	Adult Population Base (1960)	Number of First Admissions to:				First Admission Rate/100,000 Adult Population			
		All Facilities	State Hosp.	Psych. Wards of Gen. Hosp.	Private Mental Hosp.	All Facilities	State Hosp.	Psych. Wards of Gen. Hosp.	Private Mental Hosp.
60	29,111	52	17	20	15	178.6	58.4	68.7	51.5
61	47,276	69	27	25	17	146.0	57.1	52.9	36.0
62	10,464	14	3	9	2	133.8	28.7	86.0	19.1
63	21,998	26	4	15	7	118.2	18.2	68.2	31.8
64	12,801	17	1	12	4	132.8	7.8	93.7	31.2
65	19,437	20	1	15	4	102.9	5.1	77.2	20.6
66	40,972	58	4	37	17	141.6	9.8	90.3	41.5
67	42,601	63	21	31	11	147.9	49.3	72.8	25.8
68	63,352	52	27	16	9	82.1	42.6	25.3	14.2
69	45,310	24	12	9	3	53.0	26.5	19.9	6.6
70	13,350	29	1	25	3	217.2	7.5	187.3	22.5
71	46,535	68	13	42	13	146.1	27.9	90.3	27.9
72	18,024	32	0	27	5	177.5	0.0	149.8	27.7
73	21,813	29	2	17	10	132.9	9.2	77.9	45.8
74	14,433	19	0	15	4	131.6	0.0	103.9	27.7
75	19,381	21	5	13	3	108.4	25.8	67.1	15.5

INDEX